Advance Praise for

All Children Are All Our Children

"Accessibly written with sharp-as-nails political analysis, in *All Children Are All Our Children*, long-time teacher and education activist Doug Selwyn indicts the inhumanity of corporate education reform while righteously arguing that healthy schools start with healthy communities and healthy kids. If you are interested in understanding how to really fix our schools, read this book."

—Wayne Au, Professor in the School of Educational Studies at the University of Washington Bothell and editor & author at *Rethinking Schools*

"Doug Selwyn has taught K–12 in diverse settings, as well as teachers at the university level. This book demonstrates a level of critical thinking that is missing from what is taught in our schools. He is the caring kind of teacher you want for your children and all our children. Power and politics, especially corporate capitalism, stand at the root of the problem in our dysfunctional education system, which reflects our failing society. Children appear to be the enemy and schools the prisons. Selwyn looks upstream at root causes of the problems. He speaks truth about power and presents steps towards a solution. We can deschool society and bring in student-centered learning as other nations have done. This requires that we get to know our students and their home situations. Working on the challenges he presents will make us healthy and wiser."

—Stephen Bezruchka, Senior Lecturer of Health Services and Senior Lecturer of Global Health at the University of Washington

"Doug Selwyn takes a wide-angle view of the U.S. educational system, allowing the reader to see how many variables in our imperfect society impact our students' education, health, and happiness. He poses the uncomfortable question of whether we truly care for all our children and pushes us to reflect on our own compliance, lack of action, and even ignorance of the big picture. As a former student of Dr. Selwyn and now a classroom teacher, I am familiar with that nudge into the uncomfortable that inevitably pushes me to action. His conclusion is a hopeful one: if our communities have the power to erode our educational system, those same communities have the assets to work together and begin the difficult and necessary work of change."

—Diane Dame, Teacher in Saranac Central School District

"At a moment when corporate reformers continue to demand test-based hyper-accountability in our public schools, Doug Selwyn reminds us of the broad economic, health, and environmental realities that stress students and communities. He argues persuasively that we must first attend to the well-being of students and communities and gives specific suggestions for action."

—Barbara Madeloni, former president of the Massachusetts Teachers Association

"Doug Selwyn's *All Children Are All Our Children* offers insightful perspective on the current health of children and the public education system in the United States. This easy-to-read book provides historical perspective and offers advice to educators, parents, and lawmakers on how to put children's health at the center of the conversation.

I found this book to be approachable and inspiring. Selwyn's words reinforced to me the importance of establishing a classroom community on the values that I most want to instill in students: compassion, open-mindedness, perseverance, respect, and a sense of well-being. Building strong relationships between teachers, students, and families supports diverse and healthy young minds. High-stakes testing and corporate wealth have prevented a generation of students from thriving in school, and we as a society need to confront this issue head-on. This book asks parents, teachers, and lawmakers to take a close look at our ethics and to start beginning our conversations with the question, 'how are the children?'"

—Anna Marchefka, Teacher in Greenfield Public Schools

"'What is honored in a country shall be cultivated there.' The wisdom of Plato is laid bare by Doug Selwyn as he tackles the intersections and complexities between what we say as a society and what we do. Our myth of rugged individualism, that 'success' is solely based on what one can accomplish on one's own, permeates a societal attitude toward children and, by extension, parents and educators. Rather than acknowledging child-rearing and education as a collective responsibility, parents and teachers must work in the best interests of children against policies that hinder health, well-being, and happiness. Selwyn unmasks the gaps between rhetoric, meritocratic beliefs, and policies to help us see more clearly what it is we cultivate, so we may envision and actualize the society all our children deserve."

—Rosalie Romano, author of *Forging an Educative Community* and *Hungry Minds in Hard Times*

"In *All Children Are All Our Children*, Doug Selwyn asks us 'What would it look like if we decided that the health and well-being of our children was our number one priority?' The answer is our schools and education system, indeed our entire society, would be transformed. In the tradition of John Holt and Herbert Kohl, Selwyn draws on his five decades of teaching experience, conversations with students, parents, health care professionals, social workers, and educators, and a deep dive into the research literature as he constructs a devastating portrait of the well-being of American children. But this book is not about despair; rather Selwyn fashions hope for children, schools, and society with the message that the only education for social change is action to bring about that change, and he offers us multiple pathways to follow as we, step-by-step, transform ourselves and our society into one that makes the health and well-being of all children our first priority."

—E. Wayne Ross, Professor of Education at
the University of British Columbia

"As a 4th grade teacher for 13 years, my colleagues and I often feel isolated and overwhelmed trying to mitigate all the challenges students face that impact their well-being, which obviously impacts their success in school as well. I am so grateful for this book that highlights with empowering clarity the context within which our schools and students are situated. An unfortunate reality is that far too many educators and parents have given up trying to understand or change the determinants of our students' health and well-being that exist beyond the classroom (environmental, economic, cultural factors), but Doug Selwyn reminds us what is obvious and common sense: education does not exist in a vacuum. Ignoring the context beyond the classroom is not an option for the long-term well-being and success of our students—and ultimately our society. I am invigorated to organize and resist against the test-crazed, one-size-fits-all approach to schooling and fight for what matters most to us: a healthy community that honors our relationships and supports the common good."

—Marian Wagner, Teacher in Seattle Public Schools

All Children Are
All Our Children

COUNTERPOINTS

Studies in Criticality

Shirley R. Steinberg
General Editor

Vol. 529

The Counterpoints series is part of the Peter Lang Education list.
Every volume is peer reviewed and meets
the highest quality standards for content and production.

PETER LANG
New York • Bern • Berlin
Brussels • Vienna • Oxford • Warsaw

Doug Selwyn

All Children Are All Our Children

PETER LANG
New York • Bern • Berlin
Brussels • Vienna • Oxford • Warsaw

Library of Congress Cataloging-in-Publication Data

Names: Selwyn, Douglas, author.
Title: All children are all our children / Doug Selwyn.
Description: New York: Peter Lang, 2019.
Series: Counterpoints: studies in criticality; vol. 529 | ISSN 1058-1634
Includes bibliographical references and index.
Identifiers: LCCN 2018044140 | ISBN 978-1-4331-6163-6 (hardback: alk. paper)
ISBN 978-1-4331-6164-3 (paperback: alk. paper) | ISBN 978-1-4331-6165-0 (ebook pdf)
ISBN 978-1-4331-6166-7 (epub) | ISBN 978-1-4331-6167-4 (mobi)
Subjects: LCSH: School health services—United States.
Students—Health and Hygiene—United States.
Students—Mental health—United States.
Community and school—United States.
Stress (Psychology)—Prevention.
School improvement programs—United States.
Classification: LCC LB3409.U5 S545 2019 | DDC 371.7/1—dc23
LC record available at https://lccn.loc.gov/2018044140
DOI 10.3726/b14667

Bibliographic information published by **Die Deutsche Nationalbibliothek**.
Die Deutsche Nationalbibliothek lists this publication in the "Deutsche Nationalbibliografie"; detailed bibliographic data are available on the Internet at http://dnb.d-nb.de/.

29 Broadway, 18th floor, New York, NY 10006
www.peterlang.com

To Jan
It continues to be the very best book,
beyond what I could have ever imagined. …

There is no such thing as a single-issue struggle because we do not live single-issue lives.

Audre Lorde

Civil disobedience is not our problem. Our problem is civil obedience. [...] Our problem is that people are obedient all over the world in the face of poverty and starvation and stupidity, and war, and cruelty. Our problem is that people are obedient while the jails are full of petty thieves [...] and the grand thieves are running the country. That's our problem.

Howard Zinn

TABLE OF CONTENTS

ACKNOWLEDGEMENTS

There is a cliché in the research world, attributed to Einstein (as so many things are) that says if you know where you are going at the start it's not research. This book is surely an example of that. I started out in a somewhat modest direction, moved by my concerns about high stakes testing and the harm it was doing to students, but this journey has moved far beyond testing, to touch on virtually every aspect of our society. That journey has been shaped and guided by hundreds of conversations that took my inquiry deeper and helped me to situate what is happening to students in the schools within the much larger, more complex tensions between the goals of capital and the goals of democracy. There were many who took the time to speak with me at length, and while I can't thank them all here, I do want to recognize many of them.

Thank you Allen Lang, Anita Bodrogi, Anya Rader Wallach, Azeeza Islam, Barbara Bowman, Barbara Grannis, Benjamin Fels, Brittany Greene, Cheryl Dukes, Chris Adams, Christen Averill, Christy Bezrutczyk, Diane Dame, Don Fels, Ed Mikel, Gary Thomsen, Heather Tedford, Hannah Williams, Isabel Dennis, Ishbel Dickens, Jamaal Bowman, Jan Maher, Jason Favaro, Jay Lord, Jennifer Russo, Jessica van Steensburg, Jim Dawson, John Waite, Jon Garfunkel, Kat Allen, Kim Norton, Kris Echigo, Kyle Ainsworth, Lang Walsh, Leo Hwang, Lisa Mark, Louise Kinney, Lynn Gilbert, Maria Timmons Flores, Marian Wagner, Megan Matzelle, Merri Jeanne Brennan, Mimi

Simmons, Pam S. Kelly, Paulette Thompson, Phoebe Walker, Phyllis Booth, Rebecca Timson, Richard Robbins, Rosalie Romano, Ruth Charney, Stephen Bezruchka, Steve Goldenberg, Tim Hartnett, Tom Ikeda, Tracie McCarthy, Vincent Carey, Wayne Au, E. Wayne Ross, Yong Yu, and Vera Vivante.

I have worked on issues related to high stakes testing with the group NCAPE (North Country Alliance for Public Education), and I want to thank Margarita Garcia Notario, Mark Beatham, Christy Bezrutczyk, Chris van Houton, and Kathryn Brown in particular for their dedication and passion in looking out for the health of the children. Members of the Rouge Forum, co-founded by Rich Gibson and E. Wayne Ross continue to organize and act against inequality and injustice and the Rouge Forum has been a place to find kindred spirits, inspiration, and invaluable resources.

Rethinking Schools is an organization of educators that has been addressing many of the very real issues that affect the health and well-being of our children for decades. They provide a forum, through their journals, books, and conferences for educators to communicate with each other, to come together in community. They have informed my work for years.

The Puget Sound Writing Project (now Puget Sound Writing Consortium) has been helping teachers find their writing voices for many years, and models building community through teachers teaching teachers. They have offered a nurturing place for me and for many other teachers to take risks and to grow as writers and as teachers of writing.

I was first introduced to the concept of population health and to understand the role that inequality plays in compromising health through the work of Dr. Stephen Bezruchka, and his knowledge, passion, and persistence in helping to educate others has been inspiring.

This book would not exist if it were not for Jan Maher, who helped shape order out of chaos. She is an extraordinary writer who also is a wonderful thinker and editor, and she has helped me to think through and make sense of the overwhelming amount of information I was trying to understand and organize.

Thank you to Shirley Steinberg, editor of the Counterpoints series, and to Luke McCord, Sarah Bode, and Megan Madden, who helped move the book through the publishing process smoothly and efficiently.

There are, at the center of this book the students with whom I have worked, both at the K-12 and university levels, who continue to move through the world with a desire to learn and understand, to make meaning and to find a place in the world that makes sense. I have gotten far more from them than I have been able to offer, and I am grateful to them beyond what I can communicate. It has been a great joy and a privilege to learn with and from them.

INTRODUCTION

Front Row Seat at a Train Wreck

As a long-time teacher, first in K–12 and then at university, I have had a front row seat at the slow-motion train wreck that has been public education since the passage of No Child Left Behind, and it has been painful in so many ways. I had never been a fan of standardized testing, finding it a waste of teaching and learning time that provided little to no useful information to help me as a teacher or my students as learners. I was aware that it was a vestige of the eugenics movement that flourished at the end of the nineteenth and beginning of the twentieth centuries, the assumption that there was one "right" way to do and know things, a single right answer, that intelligence could be measured and reduced to a single score, and that some students (and races) were more intelligent than other students (and races). I also knew that some students did not show what they knew or how "smart" they were because they did not test well, and some had real anxieties connected to the testing, so it was a very stressful experience for them. There was little help I could offer them, but I did what I could in the classroom, encouraging them to do the best they could and to not worry; they would still move on to fourth grade.

My colleagues and I would have conversations about the tests, and those conversations were nearly as frustrating as the tests themselves. Teachers would complain loudly about the tests and I would say, "Let's not give them." They would quiet down and say, "We'd get in trouble." I would respond, "Not if all of us say no. All of the teachers in our district, all of the teachers in the state. If we all said no they couldn't or wouldn't fire all of us." And they would say "No, we can't," so I would just walk away.

It was bad education, it was harmful for the children, but we would not do anything about it. And that included me. I continued to give the tests, excusing my actions by telling myself that it was only a couple of days, that it was not such a big deal, that I could support those who were stressed, and there was nothing really to be done. Once the tests ended we could go back to real teaching and learning and we would recover.

I became much more seriously alarmed about the significant harm being done to students in the late 1990s when my class of fourth and fifth graders took the tests. I was teaching in another school, with a very different population of students. Most of these children came from homes in which they did not speak English and came from cultures foreign to the one in which they were now living. We had spent the year in our classroom focused on what we collectively valued most: pursuing our questions, concerns, and interests; learning how to work together and to communicate as speakers and listeners; learning how to carry out research and how to make use of the skills we learned to make things better for ourselves and for our learning community. We addressed the academic basics, but we did so through projects, through materials that were of interest and relevance for the children, and which allowed them to communicate what they knew and had learned through a range of modalities. They did not bubble in any circles.

I did offer them a two-week course, "testing as a foreign language," in hopes of helping them learn how tests work, to become familiar with the kinds of questions they were likely to encounter, and to acquire some test-taking strategies. They created tests about Pokémon, which was popular at the time, and the students "administered" their tests to the adults in the school. I had hoped that designing their own multiple choice, true/false, and short answer questions; writing reading passages with related questions; and then scoring the tests when they were returned would help the students to understand that the tests don't measure or assess whether you are smart or not, or whether you are a "good" or "worthy" person, but that they measure whether you have learned the particular material that you are asked about and whether you are able to show what you know using a number two pencil and a test booklet full of circles. The students enjoyed the experience and truly enjoyed that we adults failed miserably. But that did not fully prepare them (or me) for what was to come.

These children, who had demonstrated their intelligence, their skill, their compassion, their problem-solving abilities, their caring and respect for themselves and others, their critical thinking, their resilience in dealing with the extraordinary ups and downs that many families of recent immigrant (and many non-immigrant) families face, hit an impenetrable wall with the tests, which many were taking in their second or third language. Just that fact alone, that children who could speak two or three languages were more likely to fail or struggle than children who only spoke English made clear how wrong these tests were. Watching the students dissolve into tears and sink into their chairs in utter frustration as they tried to negotiate page after page of contextless test questions sounded every alarm bell, raised every red flag, and broke my heart. This test, created by people who clearly did not know "my" students, and maybe didn't know any students, created great harm to the children in my class, to the other children in our school, and to thousands of children in schools around the state. We knew it as teachers, as administrators, as parents, and as family members. We knew what the students knew and what they did not know, and we knew a great deal more than that. We knew them, knew that the tests captured little or nothing of who these children were, but we were forbidden to say anything about it.

I decided to share the tests with my teaching colleagues, who were mystified and horrified by the impact the tests were having on their students. Teachers who were not proctoring the tests were not allowed to see them and so they had no basis for understanding what was happening. My sharing with them was illegal, but I felt it was important for them to know what their students were experiencing. As they paged through the booklets they became angrier and angrier at the abuse being done to their children. And yet they continued (and continue) to give the tests and to say nothing of their concerns for fear of being punished.

I was investigated by the state for sharing this proprietary material with my colleagues; at the center of public education was (and is) a test created and scored by a private, for-profit publishing company that parents, teachers, students, and administrators cannot see. I finally experienced no formal punishment, but the chill was in the air.

I refused to give the tests the next year, but this was handled within the school, as I watched a different class (not taking the tests) while another teacher proctored my class. This "handling" did nothing for the students, and in fact it penalized them in that they did not have their regular teacher to support them while they took the tests. Any learning the students might have done during the weeks of testing and in subsequent weeks was severely compromised by the trauma they experienced while testing, and that trauma stayed with the students well beyond those testing weeks. What the children learned was that they were not good enough, were not smart enough, were not savvy enough to succeed in school or in life and that it was their fault. The testing process made them less healthy, less whole.

Many of us began to speak up about what we saw happening, but my concerns and the concerns of parents, teachers, and administrators were falling on deaf political ears.

Taking Initiative

As the State of Washington was perpetuating, rather than addressing this crisis, I and two university colleagues decided to avail ourselves of Washington's citizens' initiative process. This allows any citizen to propose legislation by petition. Our initiative would have required anyone running for public office to take the same tenth-grade standardized test that the high school students were taking, under similar conditions, and to publish their scores in the voter's pamphlet. They didn't have to pass, just take the tests and publish the results. We would need a considerable number of verified petition signatures to get our initiative on the ballot. We knew it was a long shot but hoped that teachers would jump at the chance to see the politicians measured with the same yardstick being using to define success or failure for their students and collect signatures in their communities.

Teachers loved it, and many signed the petition, but few were willing to collect signatures themselves. They acknowledged that it was legal for them to gather signatures outside of school, but they knew that their administrators would find out, and they were sure they would be punished one way or another. We had underestimated the role that fear would play in our campaign, and while tenured teachers have less to fear than almost anyone in terms of job security, they knew that administrators could still make their teaching lives difficult. Their sense of fear was real. I had a conversation with an assistant superintendent of a district who said the same thing; he loved the initiative, he believed that testing was destroying public education, and he would not gather signatures for fear of problems it would cause for him with his boss. The same held true for school board members. The pressure was felt up and down the educational hierarchy.

When we were interviewed by media, reporters would inevitably ask, "Why would you want to humiliate candidates by putting them through this?" We would respond that the state and federal governments were insisting that passing the tests was the only evidence that counted when assessing whether students had had a successful education, and wouldn't we want to know whether those who were running for office were well educated? And then we would ask, if they were so concerned about the potential impact on adults, why were they so seemingly unconcerned about what the tests were doing to our children? No one ever had a response.

The initiative failed to get on the ballot; we had no money for our campaign, and our distribution plans were thwarted by the reluctance of teachers and other school personnel to gather signatures. The hard lesson I took from the campaign was that teachers and many administrators were living in fear and would not stand up, despite their concerns about what the tests were doing to their students and to them as educators. We had naively hoped that we could halt the spread of the testing mania by shining a light on what was happening in the schools and to communicate to the public that there was no educational value to the tests.

We had taken a novel approach and it did attract quite a bit of attention; many people were educated about the tests, which was our more realistic goal, but it made no difference, or not enough difference. There was too much pressure coming from the government, too many dollars at stake, and too many decision makers too distant from the children and teachers suffering under their policies. Teachers, administrators, and school board members were too afraid to speak up, and no one was listening to the students.

It made no sense. Subjecting the students to these tests was causing them harm and the tests were worthless as assessment since the results came back after school was out, so we could not review the tests with them. The students did not actually get their tests returned; they just received a score, which made the tests even more worthless as assessment. Why were we doing this, and why are we still doing this nearly twenty years later? How does this help our students to learn, to be better, more successful learners and human beings? The number one guideline in the medical profession is "do no harm." Can we honestly say we are following a similar guideline in our schools?

Getting Our Priorities Straight

Driven by my awareness of how much our current school system is creating dis-ease and perpetuating injustices for our children, I set out to research the relationship between health and education and what that might mean for the way we organize and carry out our public education. As I pursued my questions I came to realize that there was a more fundamental and disturbing question I was going to have to address, one that I never anticipated. I began to question whether we really care about and value our children, *all* our children? I started out assuming that of course we did, but after several years of research I now challenge that assumption. We present ourselves to ourselves and to the world as a society that values life, that values children, and that values family. Our actions at the national and state legislative levels do not come close to matching our words. It pains me to say this, but we have through our actions demonstrated, time and again, that we really don't care about the health and well-being of children who are not ours or who are not within our immediate family or community. Consider this response from Senator Orrin Hatch when asked if the Republicans were going to fund the CHIP program that insures nine million children:

> The reason CHIP is having trouble is because we don't have money anymore, and to just add more and more spending and more and more spending, and you can look at the rest of the bill for the more and more spending. …

This came as he advocated for a tax bill that Congress passed that, according to the Joint Committee on Taxation's latest estimate will add more than one trillion dollars to the deficit even when adjusted for economic growth and will disproportionately benefit corporations and the wealthy (Stewart, 2017). Cutting funding for the CHIP program that insures nine million children living in poverty and cutting the "safety net" of virtually all our social welfare programs while giving more tax breaks to the very wealthiest among us is hard evidence against the rhetoric of family values and putting children first.

And sadly, as I write this we can see the response of the current administration to the murders of seventeen young people at a Florida school and to shootings that have happened since, in Texas and elsewhere. Thoughts and prayers, but little action.

What Do We Owe Our Children?

The nations of the world, following the catastrophe that was World War II, came together at the UN General Assembly to sign the Declaration of Human Rights in 1948. Compelled to respond to the horrors of that war that killed and wounded so many millions and left so many children and families homeless, starving, and traumatized, nations agreed this must not happen again and that we must cooperate to find ways to live together. The Declaration said that all people must be free from oppression, free from discrimination, and free to live their lives in safety.

In 1959 the countries of the world again came together, this time focused more specifically on the rights of children around the world. Building on the Declaration of Human Rights (1948), the countries agreed on the need to recognize and support the rights of *all* children in every country. All nations, including the United States agreed that we owe all our children these basic rights to health, well-being, liberty, and justice. And yet we are not keeping our promise to our children.

We allow nearly a quarter of our children to live in poverty, to go to bed hungry, to live in substandard housing in toxic neighborhoods, to drink lead-laden water, to attend schools in buildings that are falling apart—with no heat, using materials that are decades out of date.

We certainly have the money; the United States is one of the richest nations in the world, in the history of the world, and we can decide to use our resources to support children and their families if we choose. It would mean making changes. It might mean changing the tax rates back to where they were under President Eisenhower; there was more money to support families and children and the upper one percent was still plenty rich. As Eisenhower, a Republican president and general who knew war all too well, said at the time,

> Every gun that is made, every warship launched, every rocket fired signifies, in the final sense, a theft from those who hunger and are not fed, those who are cold and are not clothed. This world in arms is not spending money alone. It is spending the sweat of its laborers, the genius of its scientists, the hopes of its children. The cost of one modern heavy bomber is this: a modern brick school in more than 30 cities. It is two electric power plants, each serving a town of 60,000 population. It is two fine, fully equipped hospitals. It is some fifty miles of concrete pavement. We pay for a single fighter plane with a half million bushels of wheat. We pay for a single destroyer with new homes that could have housed more than 8,000 people. This is, I repeat, the best way of life to be found on the road the world has been taking. This is not a way of life

> at all, in any true sense. Under the cloud of threatening war, it is humanity hanging from a cross of iron. … Is there no other way the world may live? (Eisenhower, 1953)

What would it look like if we decided that the health and well-being of our children was our number one priority—more important than test scores, more important than job training, more important than real estate values? How would we organize the education we offer our children so that they had gained the skills, dispositions, knowledge, compassion, and empathy that would enable them to lead the lives they want to live and that we hope they will live?

My research process was three-pronged. I spoke with parents, students, health care professionals, social workers, educators, and others over the past five years, asking them for their responses to a series of questions: What does it mean to be healthy? What supports health and what undermines it? What roles do schools play in supporting health and in what ways do they undermine it? How might schools and communities work together to support children and families? What are we doing that is helping, and what changes do we need to make?

Concurrently, I was reading: about health, what defines health, the elements of health (physical, social, emotional, economic, spiritual), where the responsibility to foster and maintain health rests (at individual, family, community, state, and federal levels); and I was reading about the historical and current status of our public health and education systems, economic and political systems, and how those systems have differentially affected us based on our income level, class, race, ethnicity, and gender.

Unexpected Research: My Own Story

I did not plan to get cancer when I set out to research the question of how schools and our educational system might work to better support and sustain our health and well-being. I have learned much more than I wanted to about doctors, hospitals, insurance, medications and big pharma, campaign donations and lobbyists, politics and propaganda, and all the rest, and while it has been useful to the development of the book (and my own development and growth), it was not the research path I had mapped out. It's what happened. And thanks to skilled doctors and nurses, to my profession, one of the few in the United States that still provides insurance benefits, and to good luck, my health now is just fine.

Nor did I plan to have my mother pass (she was 95 and suffering from Alzheimer's) or to have the entire contents of my computer hijacked by bitcoin pirates/blackmailers, which meant losing every page of an early draft of this book (and everything else). But those things happened as well. Life happens, and we each deal with what life brings as well as we can, in each instance bringing our wits, resources, experiences, connections, creativity, problem-solving skills, and good luck charms to the situation.

What became very clear was my relative privilege in dealing with these events. I had wonderful insurance that allowed me to afford and access the care I needed while not bankrupting us and the necessary skills and experience to gather the information we needed to advocate for myself when dealing with doctors. We had the knowledge, skills and financial resources necessary to deal with the last years of our mother's life in ways that got her the care she needed. And I had the experience and confidence needed to dust myself off after losing my material and to know that, given time, I could rewrite and hopefully improve on what I had lost. I had a stable job and home, a supportive and loving family, and enough experience in teaching and writing that the computer attack, while difficult, was not crippling.

There are some students, families, neighborhoods, and schools that have the resources they need to deal with a crisis when it hits. They have insurance, when the issues are medical. They have money, if the issues are financial (and there is always a financial piece). They have connections. They have experience dealing with bureaucracies, with administrators or others in power, with crisis management. They know how to speak the language of power and have the time, energy, and confidence to advocate in whatever way necessary. Like me, they have the resources to deal with what turns out to be a momentary setback and to move on with their lives.

But it is also true that many students and families are not so well positioned to deal with what they have to confront and can be overwhelmed and defeated by the situations they encounter. They can't take time off from their jobs for fear of losing pay for those missed hours or for fear of losing their jobs. They have little or no experience in dealing with people in positions of power, or to put it more accurately, their previous experiences with people in power were as victims of them; they were not meeting as equals, or even near equals. They do not have medical insurance, bank accounts, or babysitters (to watch the younger children at home). They do not have working cars or the time to take available public transportation to get to appointments at various offices scattered around their towns or cities. They may not know enough

English to engage with what they have to deal with, and for some, they have no documentation and are afraid to risk deportation. As a result, what might have been a minor event in the life of someone living in relative privilege becomes a crushing, unmanageable crisis for an individual or family without the resources to deal with it.

Sam's Story

I want to close this introduction by telling the story of one of my former students. Sam (not his real name) came to our fourth-grade class just after midyear. He is a member of a Pacific Northwest indigenous nation living with his aunt. Ours was already his fourth school, and his life had been a series of tragedies, crises, and losses, culminating with the death of his parents from alcohol-related illnesses. His aunt was also alcoholic and struggling, but was family and took him in.

Sam's attendance was spotty, to put it in a kindly way, his skills were at a first-grade level, and his social skills were marginal. He was often frustrated and embarrassed by his inability to read or to keep up with his new classmates, and his embarrassment sometimes took the form of outbursts or in him isolating himself, keeping apart from the other children.

By the end of the year Sam was a bit more involved with others, had poked his head out of his self-imposed shell a time or two, and had done some reading (paired with a first grader during the buddy reading sessions our class had on a weekly basis). He was required to take the standardized tests at the end of the year and, of course, failed miserably. Those tests were clearly painful and humiliating and confirmed for him the sense that he was a failure.

Sam was in my class again the following year, and clearly things had changed for him. I think the continuity helped; he was in the same class, knew many of the students, and was increasingly welcomed as a member of the class. Sam was in school and on time every day for the entire year. Getting to school at all, much less on time, meant that he was waking himself up, preparing breakfast (for himself and often for his aunt), and then walking about a mile through the usual array of Pacific Northwest winter weather. He became a valued member of the class, now as a fifth grader, reaching out to others, working on common projects, and occasionally contributing to class discussions. His academic skills were still years behind any grade-level marker, but were slowly improving, as was his confidence.

The year-end high-stakes tests reflected none of this. As far as the tests were concerned, Sam was still a failure, scoring far below the passing score. He was reduced to a number and that was the entire story. We again supported him in every way we could to recognize the gains he had made and to make clear we recognized him for the whole person he was, but he was made less healthy, less whole by that testing/labeling process. Sam was to go off to middle school the next year, where he would be traveling to five or six different classes a day, with five or six different teachers, and I knew the transition was not going to be an easy one. Sam and I strategized about this a bit at the end of the year and our family support worker took him and other fifth graders for an orientation to their new middle schools. He left our school with some confidence, some friends, and a year of growth and support, despite the testing. I lost touch with him midway through his sixth-grade year and can only hope that he found the support he needed to keep building his health and confidence, but I worry that this may not be what happened, which is not a comment on his teachers. With 149 other students to serve during their school day, attention to any one of them is challenging, despite their best intentions.

I tell Sam's story because he is a student who has faced nearly every issue I talk about in this book. Deep poverty. Racism. Food insecurity. Housing insecurity. Substance abuse (his parents, his aunt). Chronic stress. Isolation, due to frequent moves to new locations in new towns. No modeling or advocates standing with him as he tried to make his way in the world. And a school system that focused on his deficits, on his test scores rather than the growth that he showed, and on the character he showed by continuing to show up. I picture Sam as I address each of the determinants of health included in this book, knowing that there are millions of other students across the country facing one or more of them as well.

So, to return to the question that has shaped my research and this book, what would it look like, what could we do if our primary focus was on raising healthy children with a strong sense of well-being? What could we do to support Sam on his journey, to help him to develop into and sustain as a healthy child, able to deal with the ups and downs of his life? What are we already doing, what changes could we make in the short term, and what larger, societal-level changes would we have to at least begin to chart a course toward if that were our goal?

Do we care enough about Sam and about all our children to live up to our aspirations as a just and democratic society? There is, sadly, much evidence to suggest that we do not yet care enough as a society to make sure that our children are growing up healthy, with a sense of possibility, and belonging. The first chapters of this book share some of that evidence, and they offer an uncomfortable look in the mirror.

I believe, however that despite this evidence, we actually do care, and that once we understand the larger picture, the impact that these larger, fundamental issues have on our lives, we can then choose to act to make change. The last chapters of the book focus on actions we can take, in the schools and in our communities to support the health and well-being of all our children.

We have recently welcomed our third grandchild into the world. Adrian is now a month old. Charlotte and Alden, our more experienced grandchildren, are six and a half and eleven and three quarters. We of course want the very best for them. We want their teachers, their schools, and their communities to be wonderful places for them to grow, to explore, to learn. We want them to be supported in every way possible as they investigate the world, as they learn more about who they are and how they connect with that larger world in ways that bring joy to them. It's what all parents and grandparents want. The essential message of this book is that I also want the same for *all* children and their families, for them to live in communities and in a society that offers them the same opportunities I wish for our grandchildren.

All children deserve the best we can offer them, the opportunity to fully realize who they are and to find joy and satisfaction in their lives. The society benefits when all children grow up able to realize and fulfill their potential, and to contribute fully to the health and well-being of all of us. It is a win-win. I hope this book is useful in moving us towards becoming a society that values the health and well-being of all children and families above all else and encourages us to act together in service to those values.

References

Declaration of the Rights of the Child. (1959). Retrieved from https://www.unicef.org/malaysia/1959-Declaration-of-the-Rights-of-the-Child.pdf

Eisenhower, D. D. (1953, April 16). The chance for peace. Retrieved from http://www.presidency.ucsb.edu/ws/?pid=9819

Stewart, E. (2017, December 3). GOP senator says it's hard to fund $14 billion children's health care program—then advocates for $1 trillion tax cut. Vox. Retrieved from https://www.vox.com/2017/12/3/16730496/orrin-hatch-chip-tax-bill

Universal Declaration of Human Rights. (1948). United Nations. Retrieved from http://www.un.org/en/universal-declaration-human-rights/

· 1 ·

DEFINING HEALTH

Lea's Story

When I think of many of the students I worked with over the years, there are some who stand out to me because of their presence, their passion, and their energy, and most every teacher can do the same without much hesitation. They seem to have an extra gear to them, a magnetism, a hard-to-define something that causes them to stand apart. While they are at the extreme, and rare, they are who I think of first when I picture students who are healthy. They help to define the term for me and to guide my search for ways to bring all students closer to what they bring to our classrooms. When I asked others to define what the concept of health and well-being meant to them, I heard echoes of my own experiences with these exceptionally healthy children. I will share a brief description of one of those students to begin the conversation, focusing on the characteristics she brought to our third-grade classroom. Her name has been changed here.

Whenever Lea came into our third-grade classroom, the energy in the room changed for nearly everyone. It was never anything she overtly did. By the time she had hung up her coat, taken her homework and books from her backpack, and placed them on her desk, she would be surrounded by several other children. Several conversations would start up at once, friends catching up on what had happened since yesterday (this was before computers and cell phones and constant communication), making plans for that afternoon or the coming weekend, or sharing something that would have the group in a joyous uproar.

When it was time to focus on work, Lea's focus was laser sharp. She was willing to ask challenging questions or to disagree with others but always from a place of wanting to know and to understand (and always done with respect). Lea was a partner everyone wanted to work with not only because she was smart and responsible, so the work would be done well, but also because she was skilled at making sure all voices were heard, whether it was one partner or several. She listened carefully to what others had to say rather than simply waiting for them to be finished so that she could talk some more.

I also appreciated Lea because she was a person many of her classmates turned to when they were struggling emotionally. She was a good, caring listener, even as an eight-year-old, and the students knew they could trust her. She had good or best friends, but she was not part of any cliques; no one was excluded from her world.

Lea was also quite a firecracker who could find wonderful ways to get into trouble through her willingness to try things, to explore and push boundaries and limits, always with a smile on her face, fueled by curiosity to see what could and would happen. And when her explorations ran into walls or frustrations, she proved resilient, able to recover and regroup toward the next investigation, the next adventure.

Lea developed wonderful relationships with the first graders she read with during our buddy reading, and they would follow her around when they could. She seemed to effortlessly shift the level and style of her communication to meet the level of whoever she was communicating with, whether it was with me or another adult, one of her peers, or with one of her younger buddy readers.

When speaking with dozens of people about health and well-being (what it was, what it looked like, and what supported it), it was clear that Lea exemplified many of the attributes they mentioned. They included that glow, that energy that radiates into the room, a willingness to try new things, an excitement at learning, a curiosity about seemingly everything, and an ability to question and think critically. They also agreed that a healthy child is resilient, able to bounce back from hard moments. Healthy children are comfortable in their own skin, are comfortable working alone and with others, and have a sense of optimism and of hope. There was consensus that most children have several of these attributes and that many children carry with them a sense of health and well-being such that we assume that, while they are not exceptional, they are basically ok. But there are not many like Lea, who hit all the marks.

The information about what leads to health and well-being is clear and has been clear for decades, though we continue to learn more. We know how children develop and mature as unique individuals who share a general timeline of development. We know that children who live in families that are loving, stable, and able to provide the basics (food, clothing, shelter); who have adequate health care; who live in neighborhoods free of crime, violence, and drugs; and who have access to clean air and water are most likely to be healthy. We know that living in environments relatively free of chronic stress and persistent toxins contribute to good health. We know that children learn best when they are encouraged, challenged, and stimulated to explore, to question, to experience, and to try again. Since we know these things, why are there so many children living in environments and in situations that are not supportive of health? Why are so many children not healthy?

Population Health

We are urged/taught to stay healthy by making sure to get enough sleep, to eat nutritious foods (and less junk), to exercise, to cover when we cough, to avoid smoking, and to live in ways that bring us at least some satisfaction. While this is certainly good advice, more recent research is focusing beyond individual health to the health of entire populations. Population health is concerned with identifying and understanding the determinants of health for an entire population so that we can then take action to maximize the health of that population. There is broad general agreement on the term based on the work of Kindig and Stoddart, who propose defining population health as "… the health outcomes of a group of individuals, including the distribution of such outcomes within the group …" (Kindig and Stoddart, 2003).

Some of the work on population health comes out of work done in Canada and the United Kingdom in the 1990s. In January 1997, the Federal, Provincial and Territorial Advisory Committee on Population Health (ACPH) said that "Population health refers to the health of a population as measured by health status indicators and as influenced by social, economic and physical environments, personal health practices, individual capacity and coping skills, human biology, early childhood development, and health services" (Government of Canada, 2012).

There is some back and forth between definitions of population health and public health but there seems to be enough overlap between them that I am using the terms interchangeably. Both are concerned with addressing the health of populations and include everything done to support that health, from research into determinants of health, actions to address those determinants, and measurements of the outcomes of the actions taken. Simply put, how do we support populations to become healthy and to maintain their health?

While the term population health really came into use in the 1990s, efforts to support the health of populations have been with us throughout history. Researchers at each period of history have had to confront whatever the challenges to the health of their community and using the tools, technology, and knowledge available to them have worked to support and maintain the health of those populations. For example, John Snow (not that Jon Snow!) set out to discover the causes of a cholera epidemic in London in the mid-1800s and discovered that the cause was related to contaminated water. His discovery helped to stop the spread of the disease. For another, Jonas Salk discovered the polio vaccine in the early 1950s and virtually ended the spread of polio for populations who received that vaccination.

The field of population health has broadened its focus to look beyond what would be considered health care when identifying the determinants of health. We now recognize that health care certainly plays a role, but that social, economic, environmental, and political factors have a significant impact in determining health as well. More recent examples of advances in population health actions range from various advances within the traditional health care field (the expanded use of vaccines, advances in early detection of diseases, laser surgery, etc.) to tobacco cessation and prevention programs, improved automobile safety, prohibiting the use of lead in gasoline and paint, limiting the use of toxins and pesticides in our food supply, cleaning up rivers and waterways, limiting the spewing of pollutants, requiring food inspections and labeling, and recognizing the role that economic inequality and poverty play in health outcomes and introducing policies that help to reduce the level of poverty and its impact.

I am looking through the lens of population health for several reasons. There are many health determinants at play and while they each play unique roles, they are inextricably interconnected. You can't address any one aspect of health (infant mortality, for example) without considering the many interconnected and interrelated economic, social, environmental, and political factors that lead to that high level of infant mortality. It also makes clear that, despite the healthful habits of any individual or family, there are many societal-level determinants of health that are beyond their ability to control. If an individual follows all of the recommendations for living a healthy life but happens to live near or next to a toxic waste dump, or in an apartment building full of peeling lead paint, or in Flint, Michigan, whose water supply has been severely compromised by political actions and inaction for close to four years, their health is affected.

If we want to understand and then address the health issues of our children and of our entire population, we must look to changing policy and to making different choices as a society. It is this most significant awareness that is at the heart of this book. If we want to support and maintain a healthier life for our children, we must change our conversations to include actions that get at root causes, rather than to pretend that we can make a politically simplistic call for tightening the thumb screws in schools by demanding higher standards or better scores on standardized tests. We can't expect schools to solve the health or educational issues facing our children without corresponding policy changes in the surrounding society. Jean Anyon once said that "Trying to fix an urban school without fixing the neighborhood in which it is embedded is like trying to clean the air on one side of a screen door," a comment on the politically facile attempts to "fix" the schools while doing nothing to address the underlying issues that are actually at the root of the problems facing the schools. She wrote that in 1997, and nothing has really changed in society's willingness to blame the schools for nearly every problem they and society are facing and its unwillingness to address the real issues that continue to worsen. While she was talking about urban schools based on her research in New Jersey, her findings apply to schools in virtually all communities, rural or urban.

My focus is on situating our ongoing health crisis and the role that education plays within the larger picture of inequality, of the complex interplay of systems based on class, privilege, racism, sexism, and on maintaining a status quo that serves those in power, to identify steps that can be taken, small and large, to begin to make changes that bring more health and well-being to our children, and then to take those steps.

References

Anyon, J. (1997). Ghetto schooling: A political economy of urban educational reform. New York: Teachers College Press.

Government of Canada. (2012). What is the population health approach? Retrieved from / https://www.canada.ca/en/public-health/services/health-promotion/population-health/population-health-approach.html

Kindig, D. & Stoddart, G. (2003). What is population health? U.S. National Library of Medicine. Retrieved from https://www.ncbi.nlm.nih.gov/pmc/articles/PMC1447747/

· 2 ·

INEQUALITY

Dr. Stephen Bezruchka (2005) began his talk about population health with a quiz addressing what he called the Health Olympics. We were a roomful of social studies teachers at a conference and were confident as we began the quiz. Our confidence evaporated, question by question. See how you do with these sample questions, based on 2016 data.

1. Ranking all countries by life expectancy, where does the United States stand?
   a. top 5 (highest life expectancy) b. 6–10 c. 11–15 d. 16–25
   e. below 25 (lowest life expectancy)
2. Where did the United States rank 50 years ago?
   a. top 5 b. 6–10 c. 11–15 d. 16–25 e. below 25
3. Where does the United States rank in infant mortality? (top five means it has the lowest rate of infant mortality)
   a. top five b. 6–10 c. 11–15 d. 16–25 e. below 25 (highest rate)
4. How much does the United States spend on health care per person compared to other wealthy countries?
   a. much less b. a little less c. about the same d. a little more
   e. much more

5. What is the largest difference in life expectancy (average length of life) between populations in the United States? Which group has the shortest life expectancy and which group the longest?
6. What is the most significant factor affecting the health of a population?

OK, pencils down. Let's see how you did.

Here are the answers:

1. No, it is not the healthiest, nor is it in the top ten or twenty. In the 2016 health rankings, the United States ranked 26th among OECD (Organization for Economic Cooperation and Development) countries with an average life expectancy of 79 years. Japan leads the world in life expectancy at 84 years. Almost all western European countries, Australia, Canada, Chile, and Iceland have a longer life expectancy than the United States.
2. Fifty years ago the United States was among the five healthiest countries in the world.
3. The United States ranks 29th in infant mortality among the 35 OECD countries—only six countries have higher rates. In 14 countries—including the Nordic countries of northern Europe, Japan, and Slovenia—the infant mortality rate is half the U.S. rate.
4. According to the World Health Organization, the United States spends twice as much on health care per person than the average spent by other wealthy countries. The United States spends more than $10,000 per person on health care and spends nearly the same amount on health care as the rest of the world combined.
5. A Native American man living on the Pine Ridge Reservation in South Dakota lives an average of 48 years. White women in Colorado live an average of 86 years, so the gap is 38 years.
6. According to research done since 1979, the factor most responsible for the health of a population is a measure of the inequality in society. The income gap is the statistic usually looked at. There are several studies showing this relationship among countries and within countries, such as the United States. The factors usually considered as being important, such as not smoking, eating right, exercising, medical care, etc., are significant on an individual level, but less significant in terms of the overall health of a population. Japan, for example, has more smokers (per capita) than any other country and is the healthiest country in

the world. (Retrieved from https://depts.washington.edu/eqhlth/pages/PopulationHealthQuiz0604.pdf).

Dr. Bezruchka had our attention as we all failed his quiz. He followed by sharing a chart comparing life expectancy in wealthy and some not-so-wealthy countries. This is an updated version of that chart.

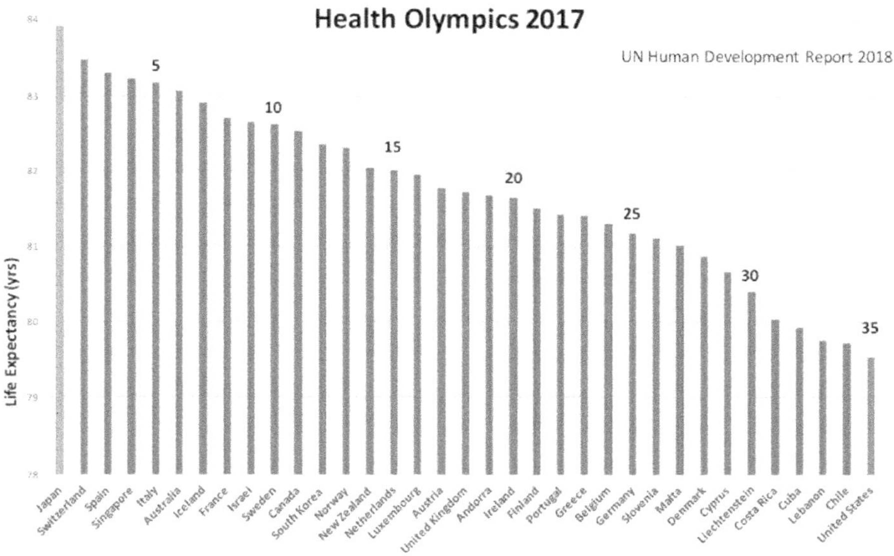

Figure 2.1: Health Olympics 2017. Source: UN Human Development Report 2018.

Those of us in the room were shocked by the quiz and chart and they raised significant questions for us. If the United States is the wealthiest country in the world, perhaps in the history of the world and if we are spending nearly half of the total amount the world spends on health care, why do sources rank us between 26th and 35th in life expectancy (depending on the source)? Why is our life expectancy below that of Lebanon, or Cuba? And, looking at the other end of the chart, how is it that Japan, the country with the highest percentage of smokers, has the longest life expectancy?

The answers to these questions are found in the work of researchers Richard Wilkinson and Kate Pickett (2009), who gathered the health statistics of countries around the world. They also gathered health statistics for all fifty states in the United States to see if the patterns in the states conformed to the patterns they found in the various countries. They did.

Their research has shown that, while individual actions certainly contribute to an individual's health, the major factors in population health are beyond the control of any individual or family. The most significant of the factors that determine the health of a population is the degree of economic inequality that exists within that population. This is true no matter how wealthy the population (assuming a basic minimum level of resources on hand such that people are not simply starving to death).

The United States is more unequal than virtually any other developed country in the world, and we are paying for it with our health. Wilkinson and Pickett found that the countries that were most unequal had the worst health statistics in virtually every category. The categories they looked at were wide ranging: life expectancy; infant mortality; mental health and drug use; violence; teen births; rates of imprisonment; obesity; educational performance; social mobility. The results were consistent. Countries that had significant inequality fared worse in each of those categories than did countries that were more equal.

Japan comes out as the healthiest country on earth, with the longest life expectancy, and they are a relatively equal country. Relative equality is a major factor in why the Scandinavian countries are healthier than we are in the United States, because they have systems in place to maintain relative economic equality across their populations. And it is why the United States is becoming increasingly unhealthy compared to these other countries. It is a troubling trend, though it is one we can address if we have the will to do so.

The basic equality or inequality of a population is a consequence of policy decisions made by a country's political, business, and community leaders. In the 1950s, when the United States was among the healthiest countries in the world, it was a much more economically equal population than it is now. The tax rate on the wealthiest Americans was over eighty percent, and the rich were still rich. Unions were strong, and there was a vibrant middle class. Families were getting education and new houses, financed in part by the GI bill (though African-Americans did not benefit from this part of the GI bill due to redlining and other racist policies and practices).

Since that time policies have changed. Unions have been attacked and weakened such that they are much less a presence than they were, and there are many fewer jobs that pay an actual living wage and/or offer benefits. The Janus decision from the Supreme Court, announced in June of 2018 has further weakened unions. Manufacturing jobs have been shipped overseas as companies have searched for cheaper labor and looser environmental laws.

The tax rates on wealthy Americans and on corporations have been lowered dramatically, and wealthy corporations and individuals continue to stash much of that wealth offshore, so it is not taxed. With that money leaving the country it is not available to fund the infrastructure and social programs that so many of our population need.

> The body of our society has been drained of its vital juices by tax avoidance. Loopholes and exemptions cost the public about a trillion dollars a year, and underreported income costs another $450 billion [...]
>
> It is estimated that between $21 and $32 trillion is hidden offshore, untaxed, with up to 40% owned by Americans. U.S. PIRG (Public Interest Research Group) estimates that the average taxpayer in 2012 paid an extra $1,026 in taxes to make up for tax havens by corporations and wealthy individuals. The average small business paid $3,067. (Buchheit, 2013)

In other words, the working and middle classes of the United States are paying for the income gap that adversely affects us all.

Income Inequality Is on the Rise

Work by economists Picketty et al. shows that income in recent decades has risen exponentially for those in the very highest reaches of the upper one percent while basically stagnating for the lowest fifty percent of the population. Quoting from their 2017 paper,

> The top 1% income share is now almost twice as large as the bottom 50% share, a group that is by definition 50 times more numerous. In 1980, top 1% adults earned on average 27 times more than bottom 50% adults before tax, while they earn 81 times more today. (Picketty et al, 2017)

Professor Philip Alston, United Nations Special Rapporteur on extreme poverty and human rights, toured the United States in late 2017 to investigate and report on the state of people living in poverty in this country. What he found astounded him, and it is reflected in his report, in which he contrasts the great wealth of the country with the extreme poverty he saw in his travels. Here are a few excerpts from that report:

- By most indicators, the U.S. is one of the world's wealthiest countries. It spends more on national defense than China, Saudi Arabia, Russia, United Kingdom, India, France, and Japan combined.

- US health care expenditures per capita are double the OECD average and much higher than in all other countries. But there are many fewer doctors and hospital beds per person than the OECD average.
- US infant mortality rates in 2013 were the highest in the developed world.
- Americans can expect to live shorter and sicker lives, compared to people living in any other rich democracy, and the "health gap" between the U.S. and its peer countries continues to grow.
- US inequality levels are far higher than those in most European countries.
- In terms of access to water and sanitation the U.S. ranks 36th in the world.
- America has the highest incarceration rate in the world, ahead of Turkmenistan, El Salvador, Cuba, Thailand and the Russian Federation. Its rate is nearly 5 times the OECD average.
- The youth poverty rate in the United States is the highest across the OECD with one quarter of youth living in poverty compared to less than 14% across the OECD.
- In the OECD the U.S. ranks 35th out of 37 in terms of poverty and inequality.

(Austin, 2017)

Inequality in Schools

This increasing inequality shows up in virtually every corner of American society. For example, our public schools are nowhere near equal, in terms of their facilities, their resources, the money they have to work with, and the education that students receive. Jill Barshay (2015) cites a federal department of education report from 2015 that shows that the richest school districts receive 15.6 percent more funds from state and local governments per student than the poorest school districts. That gap has grown by more than forty-four percent in the past decade, a result of the widening gap between rich and poor communities. Several schools on Long Island, in New York State, spend between 35,000 and 40,000 dollars per year to educate each student. On the other end of the spectrum, Chicopee, MA spends approximately 14,000 dollars a year per pupil. The wealthier districts also have parent groups much more able to raise funds to bring to the school, widening the gap even further.

Consider this public school in Detroit, for example.

> The odorous smell of mold and mildew hits you like a brick wall when you step through the front doors at Spain Elementary-Middle School in Detroit.
>
> I have been at Spain for 19 years, first as a first-grade teacher, then as a school counselor. When I first started, it was a school any city would be proud to have in its district. Today, it's the poster child for neglect and indifference to a quality teaching and learning environment for our 500 students. The gym is closed because half of the floor is buckled, and the other half suffered so much rainwater damage from the dripping ceiling that it became covered with toxic black mold. That area of the school has been condemned.
>
> Exposed wires hang from missing ceiling tiles. Watermarks from leaks abound. Kids either sit in freezing classrooms with their coats on or strip off layers because of stifling heat.
>
> How can you teach or learn in this environment? (Strauss, 2016)

Or consider schools in Chicago:

> The city of Chicago is basically turning its back on its most struggling schools, diverting funds to schools in more affluent neighborhoods, leaving the children and families living in the poorest sections of town, mostly families of color, with little help and little hope.
>
> Many of Chicago's lowest-performing schools are crumbling, but Chicago Public Schools acknowledged last year that it won't invest in improvement projects for schools it expects to be closed in the next five to 10 years, instead focusing on other schools, including those that share facilities with charter schools. (Spross et al, 2012)

And then there are private schools, where most of the decision makers (including every recent president except Jimmy Carter) send their children. Chicago Mayor Rahm Emanuel, for example, has chosen to send his children to the University of Chicago Lab School, a private school that does not have students take high-stakes tests. The Lab School has seven full-time art teachers to serve a student population of 1,700. By contrast, only twenty-five percent of Chicago's neighborhood elementary schools have both a full-time art and music instructor. The Lab School has three different libraries, while 160 Chicago public elementary schools do not have even one librarian.

Writer Mike Elk quotes the director of the Lab School, David Magill, as saying on the school's website in February 2009 that:

> "Physical education, world languages, libraries and the arts are not frills. They are an essential piece of a well-rounded education." Magill also is quoted as saying, "Measuring outcomes through standardized testing and referring to those results as the

> evidence of learning and the bottom line is, in my opinion, misguided and, unfortunately, continues to be advocated under a new name and supported by the current [Obama] administration." (Elk, 2012)

It is also a policy supported by Mayor Emanuel, at least when it comes to the public schools in Chicago. Needless to say, the great majority of the students in Detroit and those Chicago schools are children of color, many of whom are living in poverty.

Chicago Teachers Union President Karen Lewis is not surprised by the choice made by Chicago's mayor.

> The new mayor seems to recognize how school funding impacts school quality. We understand why he would choose a school with small class sizes, a broad rich curriculum that offers world languages, the arts and physical education, a focus on critical thinking not test-taking, a teacher and an assistant in every elementary classroom, and paid, high-quality professional development for their teachers. (Retrieved from http://www.huffingtonpost.com/2011/07/21/university-of-chicago-lab_n_906166.html)

Karen Lewis may not be surprised by the choice made by Emanuel but that does not help the eighty percent of Chicago's schoolchildren who come from families poor enough to qualify for free and reduced lunch. As money leaves the public schools for charters and for private schools, there is less money and fewer resources for those who remain in the public schools, which continue to crumble.

Communities with fewer resources and greater need require more, not less support. Principal Jamaal Bowman, who heads a middle school in the Bronx, says

> The lack of equity in terms of financial resources for high needs communities is a problem. They are needed at a different level than they are in other communities. You have Scarsdale, that has about seventeen kids in a class and they have all the resources in the world they need to do amazing things with their kids. We need those same resources here because our classes are too big, and we don't have enough money to teach this variety of courses that our kids need to be well-rounded. (Bowman, 2018, personal conversation)

Bowman, like Karen Lewis, does not take issue with what wealthy schools can offer their students, but instead wants those same resources for all children, especially those who are growing up with many more needs.

What We Are Talking About When We Are Talking of Inequality

Inequality can be, literally, a matter of life and death. The British medical journal *Lancet* reported that "the richest 1% live up to 15 years longer than the poorest 1% […] more than one-third of low-income Americans avoid medical care because of costs (compared to 7% in Canada and 1% in the UK); and the poorest fifth of Americans pay twice as much for healthcare as a share of income (6% for the poor, versus 3.2% for the rich)" (Glenza, 2017). It also plays a major role in the relative health of populations throughout their lives.

As mentioned earlier, the United States was a much more equal country in the 1950s, at least for white Americans, and that relative equality remained until the middle to late 1970s and early 1980s when a significant shift began. Ronald Reagan was elected president in 1980 and brought with him the introduction of supply side (trickle-down) economics and a focus on the individual rather than the public good. Reagan preached cutting taxes on the wealthy and feeding the rich; the theory was that the rich would then invest more in the economy and everyone would prosper. Then-candidate George H. W. Bush called that approach voodoo economics when he ran against Reagan in the primaries, and Reagan himself ended up raising taxes after it became clear that the trickle-down approach was not working. Instead, that excessive wealth being fed to the wealthy was trickling into offshore accounts, into Swiss bank accounts, and into increasingly lumpy, mountainous mattresses, and the gap between the rich and poor exploded.

The policies of feeding the wealthy while starving the poor have continued since Reagan. George W. Bush cut taxes on the rich (and launched two wars which he did not pay for), blowing up the deficit, and triggering the financial crash of 2008 near the end of his presidency. The so-called recovery after that crash, which involved bailing out the big banks and financial institutions that contributed to the crash, has seen the stock market rebound to set record highs. No one bailed out the poor, who have not come close to regaining what financial footing they had before the crash. The gap between the rich and poor grew even wider.

The most recent iteration of trickle down, passed by Congress in 2018, has performed as have earlier versions; corporations are taking their increased savings and giving them to their stockholders, giving out lavish bonuses, engaging in stock buybacks, and placing them offshore, out of reach of the U.S. treasury. Little or nothing is trickling down to the general economy, as was promised, and the nation's debt has once again exploded, increasing by more than one trillion dollars, which will "necessitate" cuts to programs serving the poor, working class, and middle class. Schools across the country continue to struggle to get by on starvation wages, cutting one program after another as funds for public education are sucked up into the profit pockets of corporations and the unconscionably wealthy.

The Center for Children in Poverty confirms that nearly half of our nation's children live "dangerously" close to the poverty line, and when real life is factored in (rather than formulas), adding costs such as child care, repairs on cars, appliances, transportation, health emergencies, and the rest, the actual percentage of children living in poverty would be well over fifty percent. More than fifty percent of children in the nation's public schools are eligible for free and reduced lunch, one measure of poverty (Southern Education Foundation, 2015).

More Equality Means Better Health and Education

Wilkinson and Pickett (2009) found that certain problems tend to show up in societies that are most unequal. These problems include: a low level of trust; a high percentage of people with mental illness (including drug and alcohol addiction); relatively low life expectancy and high infant mortality; a high percentage of the population that is obese; a high level of teenage births; a high imprisonment rate; and low social mobility. Children in more unequal societies tend to perform less well in schools and there are more dropouts. What matters is "the scale of material differences between people within each society being too big. What matters is where we stand in relation to others in our own society" (Wilkinson and Pickett, 2009, 25).

Harvard researcher Tony Wagner, working with documentary film maker Bob Compton, went to Finland to try and understand how that small country has been able to transform its educational system from the mediocre system it had in the 1960s to what is widely recognized today as the most successful educational system in the world. Finland's students earn top scores in international testing and there is much focus on the ways in which teachers are respected, educated, and paid, contrasting sharply with the lives of teachers in the United States.

One of the central elements of their transformation is the decision Finnish leaders made to move toward a more equal society. The Finnish government made conscious decisions to minimize inequality across the country so that there are not huge disparities between the haves and have-nots. They also worked to make sure that students are getting equivalent educational experiences no matter what school they are in, no matter what their family's income level or situation. Child poverty in Finland is under five percent; in the United States it is over twenty percent (OECD Family Database, 2017). Every school has equally educated teachers and equivalent facilities, with equivalent resources, equivalent class sizes, and equal expectations for the education that each student will receive, a sharp contrast with the United States. Finland's approach is based on the philosophy that

> [...] all pupils can learn if they are given proper opportunities and support, that understanding of and learning through human diversity is an important educational goal, and that schools should function as small-scale democracies, just as John Dewey had insisted decades before.
>
> New *peruskoulu* (the Finnish educational system) therefore required that teachers employ alternative instructional methods, design learning environments that enable differentiated learning for different pupils and perceive teaching as a high profession. (Sahlberg, 2011, 23)

Wilkinson and Pickett put it this way: "The best way of responding to the harm done by high levels of inequality would be to reduce inequality itself. Rather than requiring anti-anxiety drugs in the water supply [...] reducing inequality would increase the well-being and quality of life for all of us" (Wilkinson and Pickett, 2009, 33).

Within this broad category of inequalities are three significant areas that I will examine a bit more deeply in terms of the impact they have on the lives and health of our population: poverty, race, and gender. There is clearly overlap, but each contributes to the increasing inequality that we are experiencing as a population and contributes to the decreasing level of health of our population.

Poverty

"Why is Jason in the hospital?"
"Because he has a bad infection in his leg."
"But why does he have an infection?"
"Because he has a cut on his leg and it got infected."
"But why does he have a cut on his leg?"
"Because he was playing in the junk yard next to his apartment building and there was some sharp, jagged steel there that he fell on."

> "But why was he playing in a junk yard?"
> "Because his neighborhood is kind of run down. A lot of kids play there and there is no one to supervise them."
> "But why does he live in that neighborhood?"
> "Because his parents can't afford a nicer place to live."
> "But why can't his parents afford a nicer place to live?"
> "Because his Dad is unemployed, and his Mom is sick."
> "But why is his Dad unemployed?"
> "Because he doesn't have much education and he can't find a job."
> "But why ...?" (Government of Canada, n.d.)

The statistics around poverty in the United States are stunning. According to the National Center for Children in Poverty (NCCP), approximately 15 million children (twenty-one percent of all children in the United States) officially live in poverty, though NCCP says that "on average, families need an income of about twice that level to cover basic expenses. Using this standard, 43% of children live in low-income families" (NCCP, 2017).

Poor children are also significantly affected by America's housing crisis. Around twenty-one percent of persons experiencing homelessness are children.

Poverty and Schools

Jane Waldfogel and her colleagues researched the so-called "American Dream," that anyone can make it through hard work and perseverance and came away with a clear picture of how inaccurate that myth turns out to be. Waldfogel confessed that she and her colleagues were surprised by what their research showed:

> The big surprise for us was to find that more than half of the inequality was already there at school entry. The schools are not as much to blame as we had expected. [...] The United States really stands out, not just in having more inequality at school, but having more inequality even in early childhood. [...] The kids of the most affluent, of the most advantaged parents, they're in preschool, and they're in very high-quality preschools, because their parents can afford it. Whereas other kids—those in the middle, but especially those at the bottom—are in poorer quality care, or they might be in informal care, they might be in a patchwork of arrangements—with a relative or a baby sitter or someone else. All of this is to say that the experiences they have are very much lined up with their family resources, and they're very unequal. ... (Ferdman, 2015)

This shows up in school performance from the very beginning. Waldfogel says that four-year-olds from the lowest income families, especially those whose parents have low levels of education themselves, are already a year of development behind their peers, and that's a distance that can never be made up (Ferdman, 2015).

Out of School Factors Related to Poverty

Education professor David Berliner (2009) found six significant out-of-school factors (OSF) related to poverty that had major impacts on the health and educational success of children living in low-income households. These factors include (1) low birth weight and non-genetic prenatal influences on children; (2) inadequate medical, dental, and vision care, often a result of inadequate or no medical insurance; (3) food insecurity; (4) environmental pollutants; (5) family relations and family stress; and (6) neighborhood characteristics.

Berliner found that

> These OSFs are related to a host of poverty-induced physical, sociological, and psychological problems that children often bring to school, ranging from neurological damage and attention disorders to excessive absenteeism, linguistic underdevelopment, and oppositional behavior.
>
> Because America's schools are so highly segregated by income, race, and ethnicity, problems related to poverty occur simultaneously, with greater frequency, and act cumulatively in schools serving disadvantaged communities. These schools therefore face significantly greater challenges than schools serving wealthier children, and their limited resources are often overwhelmed. (Berliner, 2009)

Berliner identified steps we could take to improve educational performance, and it begins with the health of the children.

- Reduce the rate of low birth weight children among African-Americans,
- Reduce drug and alcohol abuse,
- Reduce pollutants in our cites and move people away from toxic sites,
- Provide universal and free medical care for all citizens,
- Insure that no one suffers from food insecurity,
- Reduce the rates of family violence in low-income households,
- Improve mental health services among the poor,
- More equitably distribute low-income housing throughout communities,
- Reduce both the mobility and absenteeism rates of children,
- Provide high-quality preschools for all children, and
- Provide summer programs for the poor to reduce summer losses in their academic achievement.

Berliner recognizes that children will not be successful academically if they are not healthy. The increasing inequality across the United States means that children living in poverty, and the schools that serve them, are operating under additional challenges. Schools serving students in lower income neighborhoods are most likely to have the fewest resources in the school house. They are also most likely to have a higher turnover rate in the faculty, which means more inexperienced teachers on staff, and in many cases those inexperienced teachers come from outside the local community, so there is a significant gap between them and the students and their families.

Berliner estimates that OSFs are responsible for more than sixty percent of the performance of children in schools, which raises a question about what we are actually measuring with these high-stakes tests. And more importantly, in what ways are we serving the children in those schools when what they need most is support for their health and well-being.

Race

The question of race and inequality is complicated, as are all questions about race. The scientific community agrees that, biologically, race does not really exist; we are the same under the skin, but there is an increasing recognition that, as Clarence Gravlee frames it,

> … much of the debate falters on the question—does race exist?—because it can be interpreted in different ways. The implicit question is usually whether race exists as a natural biological division of humankind.
>
> This question is important but incomplete. We should also ask in what ways race exists as a sociocultural phenomenon that has force in people's lives—one with biological consequences. (Gravlee, 2009)

People's lives are absolutely affected by skin color, shade, and tone, and those differences have economic, social, and biological consequences. The differences show up profoundly in economic, health, educational, and societal outcomes. Those in power have used race to maintain power, for economic gain, and to control and blame the victims.

> Time and again, racist ideas have not been cooked up from the boiling pot of ignorance and hate. Time and again, powerful and brilliant men and women have produced racist ideas in order to justify the racist policies of their era, in order to redirect the blame for their era's racial disparities away from those policies and onto Black people. (Kendi, 2016, 9)

> One of the main functions of racism in the United States has been to divide people with common class interests so that they are less able to struggle politically in their common interest; and an aspect of that function is to make race a highly visible feature of public policy while hiding or disguising anything that resembles class. (Kawachi et al, n.d.)

Consequences of Racism on Health

The health of African-Americans is far worse than those of European descended peers. D. R. Williams, writing on the Robert Wood Johnson website, says

> African-Americans live sicker and die sooner than whites in America. Heart disease is the number one cause of death in the United States and middle-aged black males and females have death rates that are about twice as high as their white counterparts. Elevated death rates are also evident for cancer, stroke, diabetes, kidney disease, maternal death—the list goes on. In fact, every 7 minutes, a black person dies prematurely. That's more than 200 black people a day who would not die if the health of blacks and whites were equal. (Williams, 2017)

The current increase in inequality disproportionately affects the most vulnerable, and the most vulnerable are disproportionately workers of color, who are concentrated in low-wage jobs that provide few opportunities for economic security or upward mobility. Workers of color consistently earn lower wages and are more likely to be jobless compared to their white counterparts, and racial gaps remain even among workers with similar education levels. Nationwide, full-time workers of color currently earn twenty-three percent less than their white counterparts (National Equity Atlas, n.d.).

Race, Poverty, and Schools

There are obvious consequences to students of color from this mix of poverty and racism. Schools are under-resourced, which means students are not getting what they need to succeed in the schools or in their preparation for life beyond school. Black and Latinx students are more likely to have less qualified teachers. Elementary schools that serve mostly African American and Latinx students have less-qualified teachers than schools that primarily serve white students. Teachers are less likely to hold a master's degree, have certifications in core subject areas, and stay long term at schools where most students are black and Hispanic (Disare, 2016).

Latinx students attend the most poorly equipped schools in the most impoverished school districts (Peske and Haycock, 2006) and are most likely to have inadequate instructional materials.

There is extensive research over the years showing that African-American students, particularly boys, are disciplined at a disproportionately higher rate than are other students and that their discipline is more severe, so that it is more likely that an African-American student will receive a harsher punishment than will a white student who is being disciplined for the same thing. The Government Accountability Office, a nonpartisan federal watchdog, found "that black students, boys, and students with disabilities are disproportionately disciplined in K–12 public schools, with the disparities for black students and boys presenting as early as preschool. …" According to the GAO, this report builds on research showing that students who are disciplined in ways that take them out of the classroom are more likely to fall behind, drop out, or get involved with the juvenile justice system—all of which can result in incarceration and decreased earning potential over a lifetime (Hampton, 2018).

This is not new information, especially to communities of color that have been living with this reality for decades. Rebekah Denn wrote a story about the disparities in the disciplining of African-American students in the Seattle Public schools in 2001, and of course the story began long before she wrote that piece. When we put this information together with the impact that a failure to graduate has on health we see that these disciplinary policies have a significant impact on health. It is a public health issue.

Williams (2017) finds that much of what is behind the poorer health of African-Americans is the chronic stress of discrimination. He cites data from a survey of African-Americans, Latinx, Asian Americans, and Native Americans that show that people in communities of color experience discrimination in health care, in housing, in encounters with the police, and on a day-to-day basis. I will look more specifically at the intersection of race and stress in the next chapter.

Political and Social Power

Another aspect of the intersection of race and poverty is a lack of political and social power. Poorer neighborhoods are less likely to have political, social, or economic clout. They are treated in ways that richer neighborhoods would not be. Flint, Michigan has been without clean water for almost four years, as

I write this in July of 2018. It is hard to imagine wealthy communities having polluted water to begin with, but even harder to imagine the issue being unaddressed for four weeks much less four years.

When I lived in Philadelphia, many years ago, it was common knowledge that toxic waste was regularly dumped in North and West Philadelphia neighborhoods where most of the households were poor and African-American. The fact that it was well known did not stop the corporations from continuing their practices or inspire the city government to do something about it. Dumping toxic and hazardous waste in poor communities is obviously not only happening in Philadelphia. Incinerators burning hazardous materials such as medical waste are most frequently located in communities of poor and underrepresented populations.

Erik Loomis (2015) documents how corporations respond to an increased focus on environmental risks by placing their toxic industries in poor neighborhoods, where people are least likely to complain and/or to have their complaints heard and responded to by politicians or agencies monitoring pollution. I go into more detail about this later in the book.

Living in a toxic environment, breathing toxic air is related to the higher numbers of cases of asthma, cancers, and other illnesses. In 2015, African-American children had a death rate from asthma ten times that of white children and were more than four times as likely to be admitted to hospitals for asthma-related symptoms. African-Americans are more than three times as likely to die from asthma than are white Americans.

Democracy Now! featured a story on the Bayou Bridge pipeline that is being built in Louisiana. The company building the pipeline, Energy Transfer Partners, is the same company building the Dakota Access pipeline in North Dakota. Once again it is big money targeting poor communities of color in which to situate their toxic and dangerous waste. Pastor Harry Joseph talks about what is going on in his community:

> The Bayou Bridge pipeline is going to come in. That means that we're going to have more tanks. We can't afford to have nothing else in this area. That's just going to destroy what we have. I think they have put us underneath the bus. And this ain't nothing new. It's always the poorest, the black and the Indians or the Hispanics. They just figure they can just walk over people. The few whites that was here, they have been bought out already. We're going to be the ones that suffer the burdens.
>
> What I'm concerned about with this one is that we don't know what's coming through the pipe. We don't know what we're going to be breathing. And we already have people that are sick. People have got cancer. People are dying with cancer.

> Nobody wants to take responsibility for what is going on now. So, who's going to take responsibility for what's going to go on in the future, you know? (*Democracy Now!*, March 13, 2018)

Gender

Another significant factor in the conversation about inequality is gender inequality. To put it most simply, women have had (and continue to have) fewer opportunities in fields that are high paying, have fewer opportunities for top-level management positions, have less access to long-term career opportunities because they still shoulder the bulk of responsibilities for child rearing and maintaining homes, and continue to be paid less for the same work that men do, at this point around 80 cents per hour compared with one dollar per hour for men (though women of color make even less, between sixty and seventy cents per dollar that men make). Adding to the inequality is recognizing that the work they do at home, taking care of the children, cooking, and maintaining the house, is unpaid. It is one of the reasons that households headed by women face more economic struggles and health struggles than do two-parent families and families headed by men. When you add in the complications of racial discrimination, single-parent families headed by African-American women are facing enormous challenges as they seek to provide for their children and themselves.

Professor Austin, after his tour of the United States, reported that

> [...] women shoulder a particularly high burden as a result of living in poverty. They are, for example more exposed to violence, more vulnerable to sexual harassment, discriminated against in the labor market. [...] The number of children in single-mother households living in extreme poverty for an entire year has ballooned from fewer than 100,000 in 1995 [...] to 704,000 in 2012. But perhaps the least recognized harm is that austerity policies that shrink the services provided by the state inevitably mean that the resulting burden is imposed instead on the primary caregivers within families, who are overwhelmingly women. (Alston, 2017)

Why Inequality Matters and What We Might Do

Inequality harms everybody, and the longer we allow the gap between the rich and poor to widen, the greater the impact we will experience across society. There are steps we can take to begin to move toward a more equal society, and there are people across the country already involved in taking some of those steps.

Support Programs That Support Children and Families

We could begin by supporting and expanding existing federal programs such as Medicaid and Supplemental Nutrition Assistance Program (SNAP) which have made a significant difference in children's health and in their ability to earn income throughout their lives. The investment that society makes in supporting those children (and their families) living in poverty pays significant dividends in terms of the students leading healthier lives, requiring fewer services, and being able to live productive, economically successful lives for decades, contributing both their skills and their taxes to society.

Medicaid is the primary source of health insurance for low-income children and includes prenatal and postpartum care for mothers. The largest means-tested program in the United States, in 2015, Medicaid, with the Children's Health Insurance Program (CHIP), reached approximately 45.2 million children at a cost of $91.7 billion.

Medicaid particularly improves health outcomes among children who gained access while in utero. A 1996 study found that a ten-percentage-point increase in the fraction of children covered by Medicaid in utero reduced the incidence of low birth weight by 0.63 percent and the infant mortality rate by 2.8 percent.

Medicaid also improves later life economic outcomes. Using the 1980s Medicaid expansions, a 2015 study found that early exposure to the program improved adult earnings and tax contributions (Gifford et al, 2017).

Recent studies show that SNAP improves children's short- and long-term well-being. A 2011 study compared birth outcomes among children born in counties that were early adopters of the Food Stamp program to those in counties that adopted a few years later. Among all families who received Food Stamps, the incidence of low birth weight was about seven percent lower for white infants and about three percent lower for black infants.

Using the same approach with longitudinal panel data, a 2016 study found that children who were fully exposed to Food Stamps during the first five years of life are more likely to be healthy later in life and less likely to experience obesity, high blood pressure, heart disease, or diabetes. The study also estimates that disadvantaged girls with full access to the program from conception to age five were more likely to be financially self-sufficient in adulthood than those who did not (Page, n.d.).

We could expand Medicare into a single payer type system that insures everyone in the country while taking the profit out of the health care business.

Studies have shown that our little town of Greenfield, with a population around 17,000 would save more than a million dollars a year if we moved to a single payer system. Physicians for a National Health Care Program (n.d.) estimate that the country would save more than 150 billion dollars a year on paperwork alone. Many countries around the world have health care for all, and while they pay higher taxes, their overall costs for health care are lower because families are not having to pay additionally for their health care, and because they are getting care sooner so that their illnesses do not become more serious. Families in the U.S. pay more for their health care and get less to show for it, as I mentioned at the beginning of the chapter. It does not have to be this way.

It is important to note that the current administration and Congress are now threatening to cut back all these programs, citing the deficit. They neglect to mention that the deficit has exploded because they passed massive tax cuts for the wealthiest individuals and corporations in the country. They promised the country that the tax cuts would pay for themselves and there would be no need to cut back on Medicare, Medicaid, or Social Security, programs that are focused on helping the most vulnerable members of society. They were wrong, and now they are coming after those programs that serve the poor, even as they are planning further tax cuts for the wealthy.

Other Steps We Can Take

There are steps beyond supporting existing federal programs that we could take. Wage and employment gaps by race (as well as gender) are not only bad for people of color and women, but they also hold back the entire economy. Closing these gaps by eliminating discrimination in pay and hiring, boosting educational attainment, and ensuring strong and rising wages for low-wage workers are good for families, good for communities, and good for the economy. Rising wages and incomes, particularly for low-income households, leads to more consumer spending, which is a key driver of economic growth and job creation.

There are movements across the country to raise the minimum wage to fifteen dollars an hour. The movement started in Seattle and has spread to many other states. Massachusetts has just passed a measure raising the minimum wage in gradual steps to fifteen dollars an hour by 2023. While that raise is glacially slow, it is a step. Other states are moving more quickly.

There are states with no income tax or flat rate income taxes, like Massachusetts. Working for a progressive tax that requires the wealthy to pay their fair share will bring more money into the economy, so the government can do more to support the health and education of our people. Taxing capital gains at a higher rate would affect only those making money from stock trading, selling property, and precious metals so that most of the population would not be paying higher taxes. Right now, those making money from these kinds of transactions are taxed at a much lower rate than the rest of us. Transaction taxes on stock market speculators would also raise an enormous amount of money. They carry out millions of transactions a day, produce nothing of value, and make enormous profits from doing so, often at our expense since their actions have an impact on pricing and policies. Having a tax of even a fraction of a penny on transactions would raise billions of dollars.

Another step would be to strengthen workers' rights to organize. When unions were strong, workers were able to negotiate contracts from a position of strength, and they could bargain for a livable wage and benefits that included health care. They had more money to spend in the community, which supported the economy, which generated tax dollars that could support schools, health care, and other social services.

And of course, equal pay for equal work would enable more women to be able to support themselves and their families, which means there would be less of a drain on public coffers since fewer people would need public assistance.

We could work toward creating more well-paying jobs, especially jobs that are focused on repairing the crumbling infrastructure that makes our bridges and roadways increasingly dangerous. This has been a topic regularly raised during campaign seasons and then abandoned after elections because it is expensive and because it is one of the many political flashpoints between those who value the common good (democracy) and those who are engaged in the drive for maximizing profits (corporate capitalism). Who should pay for the infrastructure? Capitalists ask, why should my tax dollars go into funding bridges, or ferries I don't take, or roadways I don't use? Senator Elizabeth Warren's campaign speech in August 2011 is a response to that:

> There is nobody in this country who got rich on their own. Nobody. You built a factory out there—good for you. But I want to be clear. You moved your goods to market on roads the rest of us paid for. You hired workers the rest of us paid to educate. You were safe in your factory because of police forces and fire forces that the rest of us paid for. You didn't have to worry that marauding bands would come and seize everything at your factory [...] Now look. You built a factory and it turned into something terrific or a great idea—God bless! Keep a hunk of it. But part of the underlying social contract is you take a hunk of that and pay forward for the next kid who comes along. (Warren, 2011)

The country has more than enough to pay for infrastructure if we choose to invest our wealth in that way. We could, for example, choose to recognize that investing in our population and in our infrastructure is both a matter of public health and of public safety, and move money from the bloated military budget. Investing in infrastructure is a way of supporting families all over the country to engage in work that benefits the community. It is a choice we could make, a choice we could demand our legislators to make. It is a politically difficult step because military bases are important to local communities economically, but the jobs that infrastructure projects would bring would more than make up for losses due to military cutbacks.

We could also close loopholes that allow corporations to pay no taxes, despite bringing in billions of dollars in profits. Corporations are paying much less of a percentage of GDP than they used to, and that loss of income means the government is less able to fund infrastructure and other projects that would provide jobs while benefiting communities and the country. Corporations are making larger profits and keeping a larger share of those profits.

We could also institute a maximum wage, limiting the amount that the CEO and other executives can make compared to what the lowest paid employees make. It is a policy that has been carried out for years in countries that have far more equality than does the United States. The average CEO in the United States makes more than 300 times what an average worker makes, while the gap in Japan is much smaller, with the CEO making about twenty times more than does an average worker.

We can act together to move toward a more equal society if we have the will and persistence to do it. I will share in a later chapter some community efforts going on as examples of actions communities are taking toward making us healthier and more equal.

References

Austin, P. (2017). Statement on Visit to the USA, by Professor Philip Alston, United Nations Special Rapporteur on extreme poverty and human rights. United Nations Human Rights, Office of the High Commissioner. Retrieved from www.ohchr.org/EN/NewsEvents/Pages/DisplayNews.aspx?NewsID=22533

Barshay, J. (2015, April 6). The gap between rich and poor schools grew 44 percent over a decade. Hechinger Report. Retrieved from http://hechingerreport.org/the-gap-between-rich-and-poor-schools-grew-44-percent-over-a-decade/.

Berliner, D. C. (2009, March 9). Poverty and potential; Out-of-school factors and school success. Poverty and Potential: Out-of-School Factors and School Success. National

Education Policy Center. Retrieved from https://nepc.colorado.edu/publication/poverty-and-potential.

Bezruchka, S. (2005). Presentation at Washington State Council for the social studies, Chelan, Washington.

Buchheit, P. (2013, September 23). Add it up: The average American family pays $6,000 a year in subsidies to big business. Common Dreams. Retrieved from https://www.commondreams.org/views/2013/09/23/add-it-average-american-family-pays-6000-year-subsidies-big-business

Compton, B. (2011). The Finland phenomenon: Inside the world's most surprising school system. DVD.

Conchas, G. Q. (2001, Fall). Structuring failure and success: Understanding the variability in Latino school engagement. Harvard Educational Review. Retrieved from http://hepg.org/her-home/issues/harvard-educational-review-volume-71-issue-3/herarticle/understanding-the-variability-in-latino-school-eng.

Democracy Now. (2018, March 13). Critics of Bayou Bridge pipeline in Louisiana Decry State & company surveillance of protesters. Retrieved from https://www.democracynow.org/2018/3/13/critics_of_bayou_bridge_pipeline_in

Denn, R. (2001, April 17). Little has been done about racial disparities in school discipline. Seattle P. I. Retrieved from https://www.seattlepi.com/local/article/Little-has-been-done-about-racial-disparities-in-1052395.php

Disare, M. (2016, February 25). Schools with mainly black and Latino students have less qualified teachers, report says. Retrieved from http://www.chalkbeat.org/posts/ny/2016/02/25/schools-with-mainly-black-and-latino-students-have-less-qualified-teachers-report-says/

Elk, M. (2012). Director of private school where Rahm sends his kids opposes using testing for teacher evaluations. In These Times. Retrieved from http://inthesetimes.com/working/entry/13824/director_of_private_school_where_rahm_sends_his_kids_disagrees_on_standardi

Ferdman, R. A. (2015, December 17). Only in America: Four years into life, poor kids are already an entire year behind. Retrieved from https://www.washingtonpost.com/news/wonk/wp/2015/12/17/how-your-first-four-years-of-life-affect-the-rest-of-it/?postshare=1061450460230165&tid=ss_fb

Giffords, K., Ellis, E., Coulter Edwards, B., Lashbrook, A., Hinton, E., & Antonisse, L. (2017). Medicaid moving ahead in uncertain times: Results from a 50-State Medicaid budget survey for state fiscal years 2017 and 2018. Kaiser Family Foundation. Retrieved from https://www.kff.org/medicaid/report/medicaid-moving-ahead-in-uncertain-times-results-from-a-50-state-medicaid-budget-survey-for-state-fiscal-years-2017-and-2018/view/footnotes/

Glenza, J. (2017, April 7). Being wealthy in America earns you 15 extra years life span over the poor. Alternet. Retrieved from http://www.alternet.org/personal-health/being-wealthy-america-earns-you-15-extra-years-life-span-over-poor

Government of Canada. (n.d.). What Makes Canadians healthy or unhealthy? Retrieved from https://www.canada.ca/en/public-health/services/health-promotion/population-health/what-determines-health/what-makes-canadians-healthy-unhealthy.html

Gravlee, C. C. (2009, May). How race became biology. American Journal of Physical Anthropology. https://doi.org/10.1002/ajpa.20983.

Hampton, R. (2018, April 6). A new report shows school discipline is meted out unequally according to race, gender, and ability. Slate. Retrieved from https://slate.com/human-interest/2018/04/school-discipline-disparities-exist-in-race-gender-and-ability.html

Kawachi, I. & Subramanian, S. (2014). Income inequality. In Social epidemiology (L. F. Berkman, I. Kawachi and M. M. Glymour, eds). pp. 126–151. New York: Oxford University Press.

Kawachi, I., Daniels, N., & Robinson, D. E. (n.d.) Health disparities by race and class: Why both matter. Retrieved from http://content.healthaffairs.org/content/24/2/343.short

Kendi, I. (2016). Stamped from the beginning. New York: Nation Books.

Loomis, E. (2015). How corporations dump their toxic sludge in areas filled with poor people. Alternet. Retrieved from http://www.alternet.org/books/how-corporations-dump-their-toxic-sludge-areas-filled-poor-people.

National Center for Children in Poverty. (2016, March 3). Nearly half of American children living near poverty line. Retrieved from https://www.mailman.columbia.edu/public-health-now/news/nearly-half-american-children-living-near-poverty-line

National Equity Atlas. (n.d.). Retrieved from http://nationalequityatlas.org/

OECD Family Database. (2017). Child Poverty. OECD Social Policy Division. Retrieved from www.oecs.org/els/soc/CO_2_2_child_poverty.pdf

Page, M. (n.d.). Safety net programs have long-term benefits for children in poor households. Center for Poverty Research, U. C. Davis. Retrieved from https://poverty.ucdavis.edu/policy-brief/safety-net-programs-have-long-term-benefits-children-poor-households

Peske, H. G. & Haycock, K. (2006). Teaching inequality: How poor and minority students are shortchanged on teacher quality: A report and recommendations by the Education Trust. Education Trust. Retrieved from https://eric.ed.gov/?id=ED494820

Physicians for a National Health Care Program. (n.d.). Single-payer myths: Single-payer facts. Retrieved from http://www.pnhp.org/facts/singlepayer_myths_singlepayer_facts.php

Picketty, T., Saez, E., & Zucman, G. (2017, September 25). Distributional national accounts: Methods and estimates for the United States. Retrieved from http://gabriel-zucman.eu/files/PSZ2017.pdf

Sahlberg, P. (2011). Finnish lessons. New York: Teachers College.

Southern Education Foundation. (2015, January). A new majority: Low income students now a majority in the nation's public schools. Retrieved from http://www.southerneducation.org/getattachment/4ac62e27-5260-47a5-9d02-14896ec3a531/A-New-Majority-2015-Update-Low-Income-Students-Now.aspx

Spross, J., Garofalo, P., & Waldron, T. (2012, September 11). Going to school in Chicago: High poverty, short school days, crumbling buildings. Think Progress. Retrieved from https://thinkprogress.org/going-to-school-in-chicago-high-poverty-short-school-days-crumbling-buildings-52e094bfc4f5/

Strauss, V. (2016, January 20). How bad are conditions in Detroit public schools? This appalling. Washington Post. Retrieved from https://www.washingtonpost.com/news/answer-sheet/wp/2016/01/20/how-appalling-are-conditions-in-detroit-public-schools-this-appalling/?utm_term=.adfaacd79175

Warren, E. quoted in Massar, J. P. (2011, September 20). Warren tells it like it is: "No one in this country got rich on his own." Daily Kos. Retrieved from https://www.dailykos.com/stories/2011/09/20/1018700/-Warren-Tells-It-Like-it-Is:-No-One-in-This-Country-Got-Rich-on-his-Own

Wilkinson, R. & Pickett, K. (2009). The spirit level: Why greater equality makes societies stronger. New York: Bloomsbury

Williams, D. R. (2017, October 24). Why discrimination is a health issue. Robert Wood Johnson Foundation. Retrieved from https://www.rwjf.org/en/culture-of-health/2017/10/discrimination-is-a-health-issue.html

· 3 ·

CHRONIC STRESS

I was camping in Nova Scotia during the summer of 1972 and hiking up a steep hillside over the Atlantic Ocean when a rock gave way beneath my feet and I found myself dangling about fifty feet over the rocky shoreline. I hung there for a bit, constructing ridiculous headlines that would be featured in the Nova Scotia papers about my clumsy climbing, but mostly trying to figure out how not to die. I am not the world's strongest human and pulling myself up so that I could regain a foothold was something I ordinarily might not have been able to do, but at some point, I did it. I say at some point because I remember virtually nothing of that effort. One moment I was hanging on for dear life and the next I was resting on the rock I'd been clinging to, my feet on solid ground. After a few moments to regather myself I resumed my climb, placing my feet a bit more carefully until I reached the top.

My body responded to the threat of danger as it was designed to do, releasing the stress reaction chemical cortisol and other hormones into my bloodstream that heightened my ability to act in response to the danger. This response is often referred to as the fight or flight response and is what has saved us humans over the centuries from velociraptors and mad dogs and speeding cars. And in this case a falling rock. Once the threat passed, my body chemistry returned to its normal state, my heart and breathing slowed, and I resumed the climb, shaken but back to my usual state.

That's the way it is supposed to work. However, for many people, that stress response never goes away. They perceive themselves to be constantly at risk, in danger, and their bodies continue to produce stress response chemicals. This state is called chronic stress.

A disproportionately high percentage of military veterans experience chronic stress. Some soldiers remain in chronic stress mode long after they have left the war, their bodies perpetually on high alert though there is no immediate danger. The stress chemicals I experienced for a moment during my climb never stop flowing through their bodies, at great cost to their own health. A disproportionate percentage of veterans experience mental health disorders, substance use disorders, and posttraumatic stress disorder (PTSD) than does the general population and between eighteen and twenty-two veterans commit suicides each day, more than are killed in battle.

It's not only extraordinary events that cause chronic stress. Many of our population live in conditions of chronic stress, brought on by an unhealthy mix of perpetual hunger, homelessness, or the threat of homelessness, medical crises, living in a dangerous or toxic neighborhood, ongoing violence, drugs, grinding poverty, family strife, and environmental pollution. Millions of our families are living with one or more of these issues every day, without hope of change. Many communities have lost significant numbers of their young men to prison, to drugs, to violence, to murder. For many there is the additional burden/assault of daily experiences of racism, of sexism, of bullying, of the increasing threat of capture and deportation for those who are undocumented. Many women have experienced and continue to carry the stress associated with sexual assault or harassment. Many of those living in some combination of these factors are living in a state of constant fear and stress, and it takes a major toll on their bodies.

What Is Stress?

The healthy stress reaction is triggered by a perception of immediate danger. Cortisol is the best known of the hormones that are released in response to a perceived threat, and these hormones influence, regulate, or modulate many of the changes that occur in the body in response to stress. The "stress hormones" flow into the system, allowing the body to maximize its response to whatever the danger. Once the danger passes, the hormone levels return to normal and the body resumes its normal functioning.

Chronic stress, when the stress response never shuts off, can lead to a wide range of mental and physical consequences including anxiety, depression, digestive problems, headaches, heart disease, memory and concentration impairment, fatigue, and more.

When hormone levels are depleted because of constant stressful stimuli, a whole other set of negative effects may appear, including low thyroid function, blood sugar imbalance, sleep disruption, low blood pressure, lowered immune function, and inflammation (Wilson, 2009).

Stress at the Earliest Age: Pregnancy Through Age 2

Wilkinson and Pickett (2009) stress the impact that social inequalities have on the relative health and well-being of children and on their experiences in school.

> Social inequalities in early childhood development are entrenched long before the start of formal education. We know a lot now about the importance of the early years for later development—learning begins at birth and the first years of life are a critical period for brain development. This early learning can be enhanced or inhibited by the environment in which a child grows up. A nationwide study in the UK found that, by the age of three years, children from disadvantaged backgrounds were already educationally up to a year behind children from more privileged homes. (Wilkinson and Pickett, 2009, 110)

Mercer and Bezruchka (2004) say that the beginnings of life and growth are also where health begins. The first 1,000 days after conception is when chronic diseases such as hypertension, cardiovascular disease, and diabetes are programmed, and they estimate that roughly half of our health as adults is determined during that period.

Careful attention and care to infants by their parents in those first months of their existence has dramatic effects on their future health. Mothers, in particular, need to be with those infants for as much time as possible during their early months. Unfortunately, most mothers in the United States are employed and need compensation for their time away from work, which they are not guaranteed in most jobs. The United States is the only wealthy country in the world that does not have a federally mandated paid parental leave policy. A change in that policy alone would have a significant impact on the health of newborns and make it much more likely that they will lead healthy, productive lives.

Chronic stress can change the anatomy and can change body chemistry. That stress can begin in utero, if the pregnant mother-to-be is herself involved with drugs, alcohol, tobacco, violence or the threat of violence, the stress that comes with malnutrition, illness, persistent worry over simply surviving from day to day, a toxic physical environment from living with polluted water or air, living near a toxic waste dump, racism, and so on.

Glover (2015) says that

> [...] if a mother is stressed, anxious or depressed while pregnant, her child is at increased risk for having a range of problems, including emotional problems, ADHD, conduct disorder and impaired cognitive development [...] Both altered brain structure and function have been shown to be associated with prenatal stress. (Glover, 2015)

Research shows children who experienced early stress "are more likely to be socially isolated, spend time in jail, and develop psychological disorders including anxiety and depression" (Harms, 2018).

Harms and colleagues found that "children exposed to early stress might have trouble learning how to achieve positive outcomes in their lives, like doing well in school or making friends … and end up with higher risks for mental health problems like depression" (2018).

Physician Stephen Bezruchka says that

> The socioeconomic gradient found in health status appears very early in life. Infant and child disease outcomes are related to the socioeconomic status of the parents: Children of lower socioeconomic status are more likely to be ill and die. [...] A child who grows up in poverty has worse health in adulthood than a child not growing up in poverty. (Bezruchka, 2015, 210)

Race and Stress

The history of people of color living in the United States is a nearly unbroken story of discrimination, displacement, economic struggles, assault, imprisonment, and murder. The stories differ in details and size, but the basic message has been essentially the same in each case: we don't want you here, we (whites) are the superior race, and we have the right to do what we want, to take what we want, to have dominion over you. The results have been catastrophic, with millions losing their homes, their families, their health, and their lives as a result of policies carried out by the white majority, who often justified their actions by either the courts or their religious texts.

What we are seeing take place on our borders as I write this (June 2018), with the government forcibly taking children away from their families who have come to the United States to legally seek asylum and placing those children in cages while claiming both legal and biblical authority to do so, provides horrifying evidence that white supremacy continues to guide the policies of the government. The president ran a campaign based on racial hatred, and his administration is clearly dominated by those who are aligned with him. The stress level on communities of color (and to a lesser extent on most everyone) has risen significantly.

The American Psychological Association (APA) has prepared a fact sheet on the stresses experienced by people of color in the United States. They briefly outline various sources of stress that lead to health disparities among racial and ethnic groups. Their identified sources include:

- Perceived discrimination (i.e., workplace-, gender-, race/ethnicity-, and sexual orientation-based), has been found to be a key factor in chronic stress-related health disparities among ethnic/racial and other minority groups.
- Socioeconomic status and environmental stress has been found to contribute to many health disparities among ethnic/racial groups.
- Acculturative stress refers to the feeling of tension and anxiety that accompanies efforts to adapt to the orientation and values of dominant culture.
- Daily stress, associated with lower social position and poor family functioning, can lead to adverse health outcomes.
- Long-term poverty and family stress were strongly associated with less physical mobility and cognitive functioning at older ages in African-American women.

  (APA, n.d.)

People of color are under attack in the United States in 2018. Black men and women are being murdered by police. Millions are in prison. Most people in communities of color know someone who has been either killed or jailed, leaving a huge gap in their family and in the community. Latinx workers, some of whom are undocumented and have come to this country/been brought to this country to work in the agricultural industry, are terrified of being rounded up by ICE and deported. Muslims have been beaten, seen their mosques vandalized and/or destroyed, denied entry to the country through a governmental travel ban, and harassed and threatened. A disproportionate percentage of people of color are experiencing chronic stress due to the policies and actions of the government and many white supremacists who feel emboldened by their friends in the administration.

Schools, Race, and Stress

Schools are also a source of a disproportionate level of stress for many students of color. A study done at Northwestern University found that

> The physiological response to race-based stressors—be it perceived racial prejudice, or the drive to outperform negative stereotypes—leads the body to pump out more stress hormones in adolescents from traditionally marginalized groups. This biological reaction to race-based stress is compounded by the psychological response to discrimination or the coping mechanisms youngsters develop to lessen the distress. What emerges is a picture of black and Latin[x] students whose concentration, motivation, and, ultimately, learning is impaired by unintended and overt racism. (Anderson, 2016)

Students of color face many pressures at school: they rarely have a teacher or counselor who share either their race or culture; they are often one of very few students of color in their classes, or perhaps in the school; they are more likely to be working with teachers who are in their first year or years of teaching, and a higher percentage of these teachers are teaching out of their certificate areas; they are disciplined more often and more harshly than their white peers for the same offenses or actions; their families are less likely to feel comfortable advocating for them and are less likely to be "heard" when they do advocate. Students of color who focus on succeeding academically by doing things according to the white, middle class road map that governs the march through schools are often accused by their peers of "acting white," meaning that they are alienated by their own communities. In addition, the content they encounter, especially in their history classes, tells a Eurocentric version of the "settling" and "civilizing" of America that minimizes the violence and injustice of that history and rarely presents the points of view of people of color in their own words. Students of color have heard these policies justified by white politicians who have called them savages, rapists, uncivilized, feeble minded, dangerous beasts, who are inferior to whites. Hearing the lies, the racist telling of history that essentially blames their ancestors for what was done to them adds a layer of stress and pain that they must face every day.

There is an increase in incidents of racial discrimination and harassment around the country, and this has shown up in the schools as well.

> Data from the United States Department of Education's civil rights division shows a significant increase in racial harassment complaints in schools in 2017, nearly a 25 percent increase from the previous year. [...] Preliminary police data show that the number of hate crimes in major American cities rose for the third consecutive year in 2017, driven by attacks on Jews, Muslims, African Americans, and LGBT people.
>
> Many teachers also have seen an increase in hateful language and attitudes towards marginalized student groups. Evidence shows that racial discrimination in school negatively affects students' ability to learn. (EJI, 2018)

Gender and Stress

It is also an increasingly stressful time for women. The Declaration of Independence declares that all men are created equal, which as we know only meant white men with land; women were not even worthy of mention. It was assumed they were not equal: they couldn't own land, they couldn't vote; they were essentially the property of their men. They had no standing before the law, they were excluded from most work outside the home and were assumed to serve at the pleasure of their husbands.

Women have slowly gained rights, but only after significant struggle and at great cost. After decades of protest and organizing they gained the right to vote in 1920, to make choices about their health and bodies in 1973, and to have equal access and opportunity through Title IX in 1972. The current administration seems intent on rolling back as many of those hard-won rights and freedoms as it can, but women across the country are standing up and pushing back. That's important and encouraging, but it's also stressful.

The levels of chronic stress that women have carried (and continue to carry) are due to many factors including economic inequality, the denial of equal rights, the glass ceilings that have existed in nearly every field they've entered, the hardships that single women have faced in getting loans and to supporting families, and to the doors that have been closed in the faces of women who wanted to do work that was deemed man's work.

Sexual Assault and Violence

An additional factor that has led to chronic stress has to do with sexual harassment and sexual assault. It is much more in the news and in the awareness of the public since the #MeToo movement and since the allegations against well-known, powerful men who have preyed on women for many years, but it is the sad truth that nearly every woman has faced sexual harassment, at work, at school, and on the streets. The statistics around sexual assault are horrifying.

According to statistics compiled by the Rape, Assault, and Incest National Network (RAINN), an American is sexually assaulted every 98 seconds, which means in the time you have taken to read this section one or two people have been sexually assaulted. This translates to more than 321,500 victims of sexual assault or rape each year. One of every six women has been the victim of either rape or sexual assault, and it is commonly believed that both rape and sexual assault are underreported, which means the actual statistics are likely even worse.

The consequences of sexual assault and rape are both short and long term. There is the obvious horror associated with the event itself and the immediate aftermath, but there are long-term consequences as well.

- Ninety-four percent of women who are raped experience symptoms of PTSD during the two weeks following the rape.
- Thirty percent of women report symptoms of PTSD nine months after the rape.
- Thirty-three percent of women who are raped contemplate suicide.
- Thirteen percent of women who are raped attempt suicide.
- Approximately seventy percent of rape or sexual assault victims experience moderate to severe distress, a larger percentage than for any other violent crime.

Sexual violence also affects victims' relationships with their family, friends, and coworkers. In fact, many survivors of sexual violence have been victimized by either a spouse or someone in their family, which has many layers of impact.

Self-Esteem

Women also experience chronic stress related to the pressures placed on them by society regarding how they look. They are bombarded with images displayed in media about how they should look, how they should act, what they should wear, and how they should be such that many women, especially young girls and teenagers, have very low self-esteem, concerned that they are not good enough. Statistics compiled by Heart of Leadership highlight how serious the situation is and how much stress women are carrying due to their perception of expectations, and that stress brings severe consequences.

Twice as many young women experience depression than do young men. It's estimated that approximately one in three young women have experienced serious depression. A survey carried out by the University of North Carolina in 2008 found that nearly seventy-five percent of women between the ages of 25 and 45 have issues related to eating, with fully sixty-five percent having what they would call an eating disorder. These women are starving themselves into depression, physical distress, and in some cases death.

Economic and Career Disparity

Women have been kept out of the paid workforce as equal contributors through much of our entire history, and it is only recently that some of the doors have begun to open. Title IX makes it illegal to discriminate against women in terms of their experiences on campus, and women began to enter medical schools, law schools, schools of dentistry, schools of architecture, and other professions shortly after its enactment in 1972. As a result, there are now more women in the professions than there are men, though they are still paid less for the same work. There is still a long way to go to even begin to approach equality. There are many fewer women in politics than there are men, with only thirty-four governors in our country's history, compared with 2,319 men. Women are approximately twenty percent of the U.S. Congress, though they are more than half of the population of the United States. Three percent of Fortune 500 companies have been headed by women, three percent of "clout positions" in the mainstream media, and three percent of creative directors in ad agencies.

Stress and Status

Wilkinson and Pickett found that certain kinds of sustained stress are most harmful to health. They found that

> Tasks that included a social evaluative threat (such as threats to self-esteem or social status), in which others could negatively judge performance, particularly when the outcome of the performance was uncontrollable provoked larger and more reliable cortisol changes than stressors without these particular threats [...] the highest cortisol

> responses came when a social evaluative threat was combined with a task in which participants could not avoid failure—for instance because the task was designed to be impossible, or because there was too little time, or they were simply told they were failing however they performed. (Wilkinson and Pickett, 2009, 38–39)

School is stressful for many students, especially as they move up into middle and high school, but for students who are low status, it can be especially stressful. Students who are low status at school tend to be ignored, teased, or victimized at school. Some are simply invisible as they move through the halls. Other students avoid them, or ignore them, even when they are presumably working together in class. They often eat alone at lunch or with others who are also low status and rarely speak in class.

But some students who are low status can be the subject of physical or verbal abuse. They may be teased, bumped in hallways, picked on by bullies looking to get a laugh from their friends. They rarely have allies, or at least allies willing to stand up with them in public, and so are often left to face the bullying alone. They may or may not be able to make contact with a teacher or counselor who can be an ally, but there is no guarantee that will happen. They may be afraid or reluctant to reach out, and teachers don't always notice them among the many students with whom they are dealing each day. The students are constantly aware that they may be bullied, or teased, or humiliated at any moment and carry that stress with them through their day.

Academic and Testing Stress

As the students move up in grades, the pressure to cover content increases dramatically. Classes move more quickly and teachers, who have five or more classes a day, have less time to support or attend to individual students who may be struggling to learn the material or to keep up. There is some degree of stress all along the academic spectrum, but particular stress at both ends. Students who are high achievers and are feeling pressure to get top grades in all their advanced placement classes, so they can get into their top college choices, experience relentless pressure that leave many exhausted and depressed. A student at an elite school in the Chicago area wrote about the stress for students aiming at college, at pleasing parents, and meeting expectations.

> "At Naperville North there is one path to success," Tessa wrote in the piece. "From the age of 13, every prospective Naperville North student understands that this path makes no exceptions, and those who wander off or fall behind are left

for failure. Everyone here understands that there is no worse fate than failure." (Cullotta et al, 2017)

For students at the other end of the academic spectrum, there is enormous pressure to keep up with the relentless pace of a coverage-based curriculum that has no time to linger. Students who need more time to process information, who are learning in a second language, who have learning challenges, or who want to go deeper or to question the material presented in class find the train won't wait for them, and it is one of the reasons that students who learn and process information differently than the traditional text and questions approach are among those who drop out rather than face the daily struggle to keep up.

Dropping out is a health risk, a determinant of health. "High school graduation is the social determinant that most strongly predicts long-term health. Students who do not graduate high school on time are less likely to attain higher education, practice health-promoting behaviors, earn living wages or access social capital" (APHA, 2018).

The Impact of Chronic Stress on Students

When I look at a list of potential consequences from chronic stress that includes sleep disruption, lower immune function, fatigue, brain fog, and blood sugar imbalances, I am "seeing" students I have worked with over the years, many of whom lived in toxic, perpetually stressful situations, and wondering now, as I did then, how they even managed to come to school and learn what they did. I've told some of Sam's story at the beginning of the book, but he was just one of many students who struggled to find hope and safety in the midst of significant daily challenges.

When we add the stress that has come with the hyper-focus on testing since No Child Left Behind, the impact on children has increased dramatically to where it is now at a higher level than is the stress of adults, a significant change in recent years (Bethune, 2014).

In addition to academic pressure, the focus on testing and a standardized curriculum tends to discount the social and emotional support that students need. When academics and performance on testing take precedence over everything else that happens at school, the stress levels will continue to rise, for students and teachers alike, and learning and student health will continue to be compromised.

The students in my classes, whose story I told briefly in the introduction, were most vulnerable to the highest levels of harmful stress; they were low in social and economic status, coming from families that struggled to survive economically and socially in a community that did not recognize or fully welcome them; they were being asked to do an impossible task in an inadequate amount of time for an extended stretch of days; and they were being judged on their ability to do these tasks. They were facing an education establishment that was administering the tests knowing that a high percentage of students including many of the students in my class were going to fail, by design.

When I was investigated by the state for sharing the tests with my colleagues, I was interviewed by someone in the district, representing the state. I was accompanied by a union representative; both of us had to sign nondisclosure forms just to look at the test booklet instructions (which otherwise I would not be allowed to see). One of the test booklet instructions includes guidance about what to do if a student throws up on the test (put it in a plastic bag and send it to someone at the state department of education). I can't find the precise instructions from the WASL test of 1999, but here are the instructions for what to do if this situation occurs in Ohio:

> A student who becomes ill and vomits on his or her test booklet or answer document and is able to continue the test should be given a new test booklet or answer document so that he or she can continue. Later, the student's responses and demographic information must be transcribed into the new test booklet or answer document, which will be the copy of the test to be scored. The soiled test booklet or answer document should be placed in a zip-lock bag with the barcode written on the zip-lock bag and returned to the DTC with the unused materials ... Do NOT return the soiled test materials to Pearson. (Jones, 2015)

What kind of people set up a system that assumes it likely that at least some students are going to be so upset by what they are required to do that they vomit? And I confess it was tempting to send dozens of bags of vomit-covered test booklets to the testing office.

References

American Psychological Association. (n.d.). Fact sheet: Health disparities and stress. Retrieved from http://www.apa.org/topics/health-disparities/fact-sheet-stress.aspx

Anderson, M. D. (2016, October 11). How the stress of racism affects learning. The Atlantic. Retrieved from https://www.theatlantic.com/education/archive/2016/10/how-the-stress-of-racism-affects-learning/503567/

APHA. (2018, November).Chronic stress and the risk of high school dropout. American Public Health Association. Retrieved from http://www.schoolbasedhealthcare.org/-/media/files/pdf/sbhc/chronic_stress.ashx?la=en&hash=F5FB7AF535D2CDA4CBC81236DBCE6580B53607E4

Bethune, S. (2014, April). Teen stress rivals that of adults. American Psychological Association Stress in America survey. Retrieved from http://www.apa.org/monitor/2014/04/teen-stress.aspx

Bezruchka, S. (2015). Early life or early death: Support for child health lasts a lifetime. International Journal of Child, Youth and Family Studies 6(2): 204–229. Retrieved from https://contactwellnehs.org/wp-content/uploads/2015/03/BezruchkaEarlyLifeEarlyDeath15.pdf

Cullotta, K. A., Berkowitze, K., Fornek, K., & Baker, S. (2017, November 13). No worse fate than failure': How pressure to keep up is overwhelming students in elite districts. Chicago Tribune. Retrieved from http://www.chicagotribune.com/suburbs/anxietyhigh/ct-teen-anxiety-part-one-tl-1116-20171120-story.html

Equal Justice Initiative. (2018, March 9). Racial harassment in schools surged in 2017. EJI. Retrieved from https://eji.org/news/racial-harassment-schools-surged-2017

Glover, V. (2015). Prenatal stress and its effects on the fetus and the child: Possible underlying biological mechanisms. Advances in neurobiology. 10. 269–83. 10.1007/978-1-4939-1372-5_13.

Harms, M. (2018, June 20). Extreme stress during childhood can hurt social learning for years to come. The Conversation. Retrieved from https://theconversation.com/extreme-stress-during-childhood-can-hurt-social-learning-for-years-to-come-96884

Heart of Leadership. (n.d.). Statistics on girls & women's self esteem, pressures & leadership. Retrieved from http://www.heartofleadership.org/statistics/

Jones, E. (2015). Please don't vomit on your test booklet. Valley Torah High School blog. Retrieved from https://blog.vths.org/2015/05/13/please-dont-vomit-on-your-test-booklet/

Mercer, M. A. & Bezruchka, S. (2004). The lethal divide: How economic inequality affects health. In Sickness and wealth: The corporate assault on global health. Fort, M., Mercer, M. A., & Gish, O. (Eds). Cambridge, MA: South End Press.

Rape, Assault, and Incest National Network. (n.d.). Statistics. Retrieved from https://www.rainn.org/

Wilkinson, R. & Pickett, K. (2009). The spirit level: Why greater equality makes societies stronger. New York: Bloomsbury.

Wilson, J. L. (2009, August). Cortisol and adrenal function. Adrenal fatigue.org.

· 4 ·

ENVIRONMENTAL FACTORS

It seems that everywhere we turn there is an area of the earth experiencing a disaster of one variety or another, or just recovering from one. Storms that used to be called "storms of the century," which approximated their frequency, are happening much more often and much more intensely, and the health and future of life on the planet are becoming very real questions. It doesn't just seem worse; it is worse.

According to the UN's disaster monitoring system, America sits alongside China and India in suffering the greatest number of natural disasters globally between 1995 and 2015. These include earthquakes, storms, floods, and heat waves. Since 1970, the number of disasters worldwide has more than quadrupled to around 400 a year. September of 2017 was the most active hurricane month in history.

The last several years have also brought other kinds of disasters, more directly associated with human actions, ranging from poisoned water in Flint and other cities across the country, record setting forest fires, mud slides, to oil spills associated with pipelines, offshore drilling, and transportation accidents.

Environmental risk is also high for people simply living their daily lives if those lives are located near toxic waste facilities, incinerators, super fund sites, or locations where industry has deposited its waste. People living in communities on sea level islands or on coastlines are losing land to erosion, and some are about to lose their homes due to flooding. For them, climate change is not a political or scientific theory; it is a reality that is literally lapping at their doors. Families who live in environmentally toxic neighborhoods or towns are at increased risk of developing debilitating and, in some cases, life-threatening diseases, and schools that are working with children growing up in these toxic environments are working with children whose learning potentials may well be compromised, a situation that is clearly beyond the control of any teacher or school. I will briefly present a few examples of the ways in which a toxic environment has an impact on the learning of children but, more importantly, has an impact on the health of the entire populations living in those cities, towns, and regions.

Flint, Michigan

The politically appointed city manager of Flint, Michigan, made the decision to change the source of that city's drinking water from the Detroit River to the Flint River, with disastrous consequences. Here is Melissa Mays, a resident of Flint, speaking with Amy Goodman from *Democracy Now*!

MELISSA MAYS: All three of my sons are anemic now. They have bone pain every single day. They miss a lot of school because they're constantly sick. Their immune systems are compromised … And I know that we're not the only one. I'm getting calls from people that are so sick, and they don't know what to do.

AMY GOODMAN: How old are your boys?

MELISSA MAYS: Eleven, 12 and 17. And they're wonderful kids; they put forth all this effort to get straight A's, to get good grades. My oldest, it's little things that he seems to forget, like pluses and minuses, different words he can't—there's a brain fog that's settled on everybody.

AMY GOODMAN: Mayor Weaver has called for $55 million to replace the lead pipes. Is that happening?

MELISSA MAYS: It's still—we're still waiting. (*Democracy Now*!, 2016)

And they are still waiting, in 2018. The politics and economics around the poisoning of Flint's water supply is both instructive and deeply disturbing. General Motors was born in Flint and maintained a major presence there for decades. Flint was known as "Vehicle City," and tens of thousands lived well on the good-paying union jobs located in factories all over town. When the company pulled out of Flint, moving some of its facilities to the suburbs, some to other countries, the tax base collapsed, leaving behind a population with no work and no money to pay to keep the infrastructure going.

As bad as things are in Flint, it is not the only city experiencing these issues. This is from a story researched by Reuters:

> Flint is just one of thousands of towns and cities across the Midwest, the so-called Rust Belt, left behind by industry and the economic recovery enjoyed by those on Wall Street. Many of these towns are now inhabited by a largely African American population originally drawn by well-paying industry jobs and now too poor or too settled to consider moving and suffering as the infrastructure of their towns collapse around them. Flint is by no means the only town with high lead levels; in fact, it is not even among the most polluted. (Pell and Schneyer, 2016)

In all, Reuters found nearly 3,000 areas with recently recorded lead poisoning rates at least double those in Flint during the peak of that city's contamination crisis. And more than 1,100 of these communities had a rate of elevated blood tests at least four times higher.

> Like Flint, many of these localities are plagued by legacy lead: crumbling paint, plumbing, or industrial waste left behind. Unlike Flint, many have received little attention or funding to combat poisoning. (Pell and Schneyer, 2016)

The story of Flint is different only because it became known to the public. It brings together many elements that conspire to compromise the health of populations: inequality, poverty, racism, governmental policy, and business. This mix leaves populations desperate, ill, and without hope.

The governments of various towns, cities, and states claim to monitor water pollution, but in many cases they are not being honest about that. Marc Edwards, the scientist who first uncovered the crisis in Flint, described water testing in some of America's largest cities as an "outrage."

> "They make lead in water low when collecting samples for EPA compliance, even as it poisons kids who drink the water," Edwards, a Virginia Tech scientist, said. "Clearly, the cheating and lax enforcement are needlessly harming children all over the United States. If they cannot be trusted to protect little kids from lead in drinking water, what on Earth can they be trusted with? Who amongst us is safe?" (Edwards, quoted in Pierce, 2016)

Lead Poisoning

Lead poisoning is the most harmful and most often mentioned of the pollutants coming through the pipes in Flint and those other cities and towns, so what is it and why is it so harmful? The Mayo Clinic has posted a list of symptoms associated with lead poisoning, highlighting the impact that it can have. The list includes: developmental delay, learning difficulties, irritability, loss of appetite, weight loss, sluggishness and fatigue, abdominal pain, vomiting, constipation, hearing loss, and seizures. The consequences of lead poisoning are often not recognized or connected to lead as the cause, and schools are often having to provide extra services to support children experiencing the consequences of lead poisoning. A study carried out by Kaiser noted that children screened for lead poisoning were more than likely to be receiving services for behavior problems, mental retardation, learning disabilities, or a speech language impairment than other children attending the same school (Mayo Clinic, n.d.).

Lead is especially dangerous for a developing fetus and for newborns because of their rapid metabolisms and the speed of their growth. "Lead is toxic to everyone, but unborn babies and young children are at greatest risk for health problems from lead poisoning—their smaller, growing bodies make them more susceptible to absorbing and retaining lead." (Retrieved from http://kidshealth.org/parent/firstaid_safe/home/lead_poisoning.html#)

Where Does It Come From?

An estimated four million households in which children are living are being exposed to high levels of lead (Centers for Disease Control, 2017). The Centers for Disease Control (CDC) estimates that there are more than half a million children ages 1–5 in the United States with blood levels above the levels at which they recommend public health actions. Children with these dangerously high blood lead levels are disproportionately located in poor communities, and in communities of color (which are disproportionately poor). Why is that? Lead paint. Once upon a time lead-based paints were used on homes and apartments before they were outlawed in 1978 due to health concerns. Many older apartment buildings in poorer neighborhoods, especially those owned and operated by slumlords, have not painted or repainted their buildings in all these years and so flaking, chipping lead-based paint is present, and young children, who put everything in their mouths, are exposed to the lead in the paint.

Lead is also found in contaminated soil located near busy streets, where lead deposits from leaded gas still sit, in water that flows through old lead pipes or faucets and even in some imported foods and toys.

Corporations Dump Waste on the Poor

Lead is not the only toxin that neighborhoods and families experience, especially those in low-income areas. As I mentioned in the previous chapter, corporations have chosen to dump toxic waste in poor communities for a very long time, recognizing that those communities have little political clout and few resources they can organize to fight such behavior. Eric Loomis (2015) describes the behavior of Chemical Waste Management as an example of the practice:

> In 1978, Chemical Waste Management, a company that specialized in handling toxic waste, chose the community of Emelle, in Sumter County, Alabama, as the site of its new toxic waste dump. Corporations contracted with Chem Waste to handle their toxic waste. Sumter County was over two-thirds African American and over one-third of the county's residents lived in poverty, but whites made up the county political elite approving the decision.
>
> In Emelle, more than 90 percent of the residents were black. This is why Chem Waste chose Emelle. [...] The company dumped polychlorinated biphenyls (PCBs) and other toxic materials at the site. Despite claiming it was safe, the company racked up hundreds of thousands of dollars in fines. Such activities were common for Chem Waste. It always chose communities like this to site its dumps—Port Arthur, Texas, in a neighborhood that was 80 percent people of color; Chicago's South Side in a neighborhood 79 percent people of color; and Saguet, Illinois, a 95 percent African American area. (Loomis, 2015)

This is not the exception, it is the rule. Communities of color and the most impoverished communities have regularly become the sites of incinerators burning toxic waste, including medical waste. And while steps have been taken to challenge such corporate malfeasance, it is still going on.

> Poverty and race too often mean toxic exposure and cancer in the United States. In a 2014 report, researchers at the University of Minnesota demonstrated that people of color in the United States breathe in air 38 percent more polluted than whites. In the Los Angeles metro area, 91 percent of the 1.2 million people who live less than two miles from hazardous-waste treatment facilities are people of color. Environmental inequality is a systematic problem made worse by intentional corporate decisions to profit off of poisoning minority populations. (Loomis, 2015)

Mining

Mining has been a major source of the materials essential to industrial production in the United States and around the world. The country's factories and industries ran on coal and now run on a combination of coal, natural gas, and oil. Other extractive industries, including mining for gold, silver, copper, iron, nickel, and other metals, have also played a significant role in the nation's economy at various times through our history. There has been a devastating impact on the health of those living around the mines or downstream from rivers into which the tailings and waste from mining operations have been dumped. The current administration has made a point of promising to bring back coal, to support clean coal (there is no such thing), and to loosen environmental and safety protections that protect the environment and workers but that cut into the profits of the companies doing the mining.

What's Wrong With Coal?

There are a number of negative health effects of coal that occur through its mining, preparation, combustion, waste storage, and transport. Negative health effects from coal use within the United States include:

- Reduction in life expectancy
- Respiratory hospital admissions
- Black lung
- Congestive heart failure
- Nonfatal cancer, osteoporosis, ataxia, renal dysfunction
- Chronic bronchitis, asthma attacks, etc.
- Loss of IQ from air and water pollution and nervous system damage
- Degradation and soiling of buildings that can affect human health
- Ecosystem loss and degradation, with negative effects on health and quality of life.
  (Source: Watch, 2015)

Communities living near mining operations, mostly white and mostly desperately poor, support the continuation of mining because it is often the only source of employment for the community, and mining companies threaten to leave if the residents push for tighter environmental protections and health and safety protections for workers. They are caught in an impossible situation in which their immediate source of income is balanced against the likelihood that they and their children will be dealing with the health impacts of mining operations.

In addition, Congress just passed legislation that says that mining companies do not have to plan for or budget for cleanup after they have completed their mining operations, which means that the toxic sludge, tailings, and other wastes created by mining is a problem for the communities. The health of children growing up near mines is affected by them breathing air and drinking water that have been polluted by the mining operation. Research has shown that asthma, attention-deficit hyperactivity disorder, gastrointestinal problems, difficulty falling asleep, frequent night awakenings, sleep talking, and complaints of leg cramps were greater in children living near coal ash compared to children not living near coal ash (Sears and Zierold, 2017). They are also living with family members, especially parents, whose health has been severely compromised by their work in the mines, resulting in disability or even death, which has both emotional and economic consequences.

What Can We Do?

There are actions in support of planet health that are quiet ones, such as picking up litter, setting up compost bins and recycling stations, taking care with water usage, such as choosing to not water your lawn during dry spells, taking shorter showers, collecting rainwater in collectors for use in the garden, and using gray water in the garden, and many of these actions can and do take place in and around schools.

There have historically been significant movements to protect the environment from the ravages of industry, most notably direct-action campaigns against nuclear power, oil pipelines and drilling, and industries spewing waste into the air, water, and earth. There have also been court cases and legislation that has put in place protections against industry pollution, and our cities, rivers, and air are much cleaner than they once were, but the overall health of the planet is in greater and greater risk due to the threat of climate change, a threat that doesn't seem to interest or concern those in the current administration. They have said plainly that the needs of corporations and big business to make profits are more important than the needs of the people or the planet, and so they are rolling back many of the protections that have helped to limit the damage.

Our Children's Trust

There is a court case that has been filed by young people who are suing the government for their unwillingness to protect them and their future. They began their lawsuit against the Obama Administration and now have shifted it to the current administration, which has tried to dismiss the case or to postpone it. The courts have supported it going forward and there is a trial date set for October 29, 2018.

The plaintiffs are young people from around the country, ages 10–21, and they have charged the government with endangering their right to life by its failure to act against climate change.

This summary of their case is taken from their website:

> Youth filed their constitutional climate lawsuit, called *Juliana v. U.S.*, against the U.S. government in the U.S. District Court for the District of Oregon in 2015.
>
> Their complaint asserts that, through the government's affirmative actions that cause climate change, it has violated the youngest generation's constitutional rights to life, liberty, and property, as well as failed to protect essential public trust resources,
>
> The fossil fuel industry initially intervened in the case as defendants, joining the U.S. government in trying to have the case dismissed, but they have since withdrawn from the case.
>
> The ninth circuit has rejected the government's attempts to have the case dismissed, but they have been able to delay the court date, which is now scheduled for October 2018.
>
> For more information on Our Children's Trust and their case, go to their website at https://www.ourchildrenstrust.org/us/federal-lawsuit.

References

Centers for Disease Control. (2017). Lead. Retrieved from https://www.cdc.gov/nceh/lead/

Democracy Now. (2016, February 17). "Thirsty for democracy: The poisoning of an American city": Complete Democracy Now! Special on Flint. Retrieved from https://www.democracynow.org/2016/2/17/thirsty_for_democracy_the_poisoning_of_an

Kids Health. (n.d.). Lead poisoning. Retrieved from http://kidshealth.org/en/parents/lead-poisoning.html#

Loomis, E. (2015). Out of sight: The long and disturbing story of corporations outsourcing catastrophe. New York: New Press.

Mayo Clinic. (n.d.). Lead poisoning. Retrieved from http://www.mayoclinic.org/diseases-conditions/lead-poisoning/symptoms-causes/dxc-20275054

Our Children's Trust. (n.d.). Juliana v. U.S.-Climate Lawsuit. Retrieved from https://www.ourchildrenstrust.org/

Pell, M. B. & Schneyer, J. (2016, December 19). The thousands of U.S. locales where lead poisoning is worse than in Flint. Retrieved from http://www.reuters.com/investigates/special-report/usa-lead-testing/

Pierce, C. P. (2016, June 2). The nation's poisonous water problem is far worse than you think. Esquire. Retrieved from https://www.esquire.com/news-politics/politics/news/a45451/lead-water-crisis-33-cities/

Sears, C. G. & Zierold, K. M. (2017, July 25). Health of children living near coal ash. Global Pediatric Health. Retrieved from https://www.ncbi.nlm.nih.gov/pmc/articles/PMC5533260/

Source Watch. (2015). Health effects of coal. Source Watch. Retrieved from https://www.sourcewatch.org/index.php/Health_effects_of_coal

· 5 ·

CORPORATE CAPITALISM V. DEMOCRACY AND THE COMMON GOOD

When I taught in elementary I would teach a math lesson that presented my third graders with an outline of the largest organism in the world, the blue whale. I would tape off an outline of the whale and we would measure it, figure out how many of us could fit inside of it, plot the volume, research how much it ate, watch videos of it and so on. It was a pretty cool lesson and the students were totally engaged. The problem with it is that in one fundamental way it was inaccurate. The blue whale is not the largest organism on earth. The largest organism on earth is not even one of those redwoods growing large and tall in California. The largest organism on earth is a mushroom.

More precisely, a specific honey fungus measuring 2.4 miles (3.8 km) across, growing in the Blue Mountains in Oregon is thought to be the largest living organism on Earth. We see clumps of these little honey mushrooms popping up throughout the forest; what we don't see is the underground network that spans miles, and that can bring death.

> Several species of fungi belong to the Armillaria genus, which is popularly known as honey fungus. They colonize and kill a variety of trees and woody plants. The large clumps of yellow-brown mushrooms that appear above ground are the fruiting bodies of much larger organisms. They consist mainly of black bootlace-like rhizomorphs that spread out below surface in search of new hosts, and underground networks of tubular filaments called mycelia.

> When mycelia that are genetically identical meet, they can fuse to form one individual. The most widely-spaced were 2.4 miles (3.8 km) apart. The team calculated that the honey mushroom in question covered an area of 3.7 square miles (9.6 square km) and was somewhere between 1,900 and 8,650 years old. (Fleming, 2014)

I think of these mushrooms when I think about capitalism and about the issues that we confront every day. Like the small clumps of honey mushrooms that we find at various parts of a forest, issues seem to pop up in isolation, a school funding crisis here, a lack of access to health care there, an oil spill here, and here, and here, crumbling bridges and infrastructure there, thousands of young immigrant children separated from their families and placed in cages, over there, a lessening of insurance coverage there, an invasion of an oil-rich country (for its own good) there, a roll back of environmental protections everywhere. Each of these events is experienced as a separate, isolated event but, like the honey mushrooms, they are connected underneath by a vast network of fibers and are collectively destroying the environment in which they are growing.

If we are to be effective in our efforts to restore health and well-being to our society we do well to recognize that these seemingly disconnected events are connected, and that addressing any one of them in isolation is at best a temporary fix. It is why we can't simply "fix" schools while doing nothing about the surrounding neighborhoods. It doesn't work, any more than picking a clump of mushrooms would "solve" the growth of the fungus and save the trees threatened by them.

This chapter looks at the intersections of and conflicts between the two contradictory pillars of the United States, corporate capitalism and democracy.

For many people the United States symbolizes the power and virtue of both capitalism and democracy, and the two are often intertwined when politicians talk of what makes the country great.

> Our Founders considered themselves heirs to principles that were timeless and truths that were self-evident. When Jefferson sat down to write, he was trying, he said, to place before mankind 'the common sense of the subject.' The common sense of the subject was that we should be free. And though great evils would linger, the world would never be the same after July 4, 1776.
>
> A wonderful country was born, and a revolutionary idea sent forth to all mankind: Freedom, not by the good graces of government but as the birthright of every individual; equality, not as a theory of philosophers but by the design of our Creator; natural rights, not for the few, not even for a fortunate many but for all people, in all places, in all times. (President George W. Bush, 2001)

These self-evident truths of Jefferson and the other founders, that all men are created equal, has been held up to the world as evidence that America is truly an exceptional country, a "shining city on a hill," as President Reagan phrased it. And, as we know, those aspirational words were written by a man who owned hundreds of other human beings, at a time when women and children had no rights, or legal standing. Native Americans had no rights either and were being driven from their lands and/or murdered, and there were tens of thousands of enslaved Africans, owned by those "equal men." It was clear that the American ideal, which came to be called the American Dream, was intended for and reserved for only rich white men living on American soil.

Frederick Douglass brought this point to an audience he had been invited to address on July 4, 1852 in a speech now titled What to a Slave is the Fourth of July? Here is a small part of that speech.

> What, to the American slave, is your 4th of July? I answer; a day that reveals to him, more than all other days in the year, the gross injustice and cruelty to which he is the constant victim. To him, your celebration is a sham; your boasted liberty, an unholy license; your national greatness, swelling vanity; your sounds of rejoicing are empty and heartless; your denunciation of tyrants, brass fronted impudence; your shouts of liberty and equality, hollow mockery; your prayers and hymns, your sermons and thanksgivings, with all your religious parade and solemnity, are, to Him, mere bombast, fraud, deception, impiety, and hypocrisy-a thin veil to cover up crimes which would disgrace a nation of savages. There is not a nation on the earth guilty of practices more shocking and bloody than are the people of the United States, at this very hour. (Frederick Douglass, 1852)

Despite hundreds of years of evidence to the contrary, America still presents itself to itself and the world as a beacon of freedom and possibility, hence President Bush's speech given in 2001. It is a myth that reaches down to the lowest levels of our economic ladder, promising that anyone can grow up to be successful, no matter how humble his or her origins, no matter how mean their circumstances. It is, to repeat, a myth that has no basis in the real world. There is less mobility in America, from poor to middle class much less to the wealthy class, than in virtually any developed country on earth (Kraus and Tan, 2015). Despite the promise of democracy, where the government exists to serve the people who retain the ultimate power, the realities of corporate capitalism, the economic system that serves as the foundation of the nation's economy undermine and nullify any possibility of equality. These two fundamental systems on which American society rests, democracy and capitalism are in fact perpetually at odds, the goals and tenets of the one contradicting the goals and tenets of the other. At times through our history there has been movement towards more democracy. The Civil Rights movement, the women's movement, and the labor movement all brought changes that improved the lives of the people by both winning more rights, by opening the door to fuller participation, and by protecting the public from the excesses of exploitation by corporations in pursuit of profits.

At other times, such as what we are experiencing today, the ruthless behaviors of corporate capitalism have assaulted our people, our environment, and our basic morality in pursuit of their short-term profits, and many perceive there to be less democracy as a result. The top 1% of our population has wealth equal to the wealth of the bottom 90% (Monaghan, 2014), which leaves them wielding enormous power and influence, while the ninety percent have little wealth, power, or influence over major factors in their lives. This contradiction has led to the grossly unequal nightmare for millions living in poverty, living with little hope of living the life promised by the fine words penned by Jefferson centuries ago.

Until we appreciate the fundamental roles that capitalism and democracy play in our daily lives, in the ways they shape and determine the institutions and policies that control our lives we will be limited in our appreciation of what needs to be done to make the change we seek, and to understand how things have come to be.

What Is Corporate Capitalism?

Corporate capitalism permeates every aspect of our lives and is the throughline to many of the issues that compromise the health and well-being of our population. Kasser and Linn identify corporate capitalism as the macrosystem that shapes the values, beliefs, and institutions within the United States. They define the fundamental tenets of capitalism:

- The system prefers private ownership to commonly shared property; from capitalism's point of view, it is better for each family in a neighborhood to own a lawnmower than for a group of families to share one.
- People living under capitalism are encouraged to pursue their own self-interests, primarily the accumulation of wealth and possessions.
- Capitalism holds that, in a free market relatively unencumbered by governmental regulations, competition will work like an "invisible hand" to create the highest quality and lowest-priced goods and services (Kasser and Linn, 2016, 124)

They add that "the more that a nation has a "competitive" or "economically free" form of capitalism, the more that its citizens value mastery and hierarchy and the less that they value egalitarianism, harmony, and intellectual autonomy (Kasser and Linn, 2016, 126).

Noam Chomsky adds that these private corporations, that control most of the money and, increasingly the policies and politicians that make policy, are unaccountable. They are not obligated to open their books, to discuss their operations with the public, and owe nothing to the citizens of the country in which they sit.

> What is called 'capitalism' is basically a system of corporate mercantilism, with huge and largely unaccountable private tyrannies exercising vast control over the economy, political systems, and social and cultural life, operating in close cooperation with powerful states that intervene massively in the domestic economy and international society. (Chomsky, 2004, 784)

What Is a Democracy?

There are basic principles common to all democracies. According to civiced.org, those principles include:

- Rule by the People through free and fair elections and other forms of participation. Popular sovereignty—the idea that the People are the ultimate authority and the source of the authority of government—is a fundamental principle of democracy.
- The political equality of all citizens is an essential principle of democracy.
- The just powers of government are based upon the consent of the governed.
- Free elections and other forms of civic participation are essential to democracy. If the People are to rule, they must have practical means of determining who shall exercise political power on their behalf. If they are to rule, the People must also monitor and influence officials' behavior while in office.
- Elections are at the heart of the practical means for the People to assert their sovereignty; they must be free, fair, and sufficiently frequent if the People's will is to have effect.
- Voters must not be stopped from voting and all votes must be accurately counted.
- As overseers of government, the People must have alternative sources of information. No single source, especially an official government source, is sufficient. Freedom of the press is therefore an essential aspect of democratic government. (civiced.org, n.d.)

The United States has a representative democracy (rather than a pure democracy), but the underlying principles still apply, at least in theory. Power still rests with the people, the government still governs with the consent of the people, but instead of voting on issues themselves, people elect representatives to make governing decisions for them.

Democracy and Capitalism

Comparing the principles of democracy and capitalism listed above, there are many contradictions.

Table 6.1: Democracy and Capitalism.

Democracy	Capitalism
Democracy is a system of government, and its responsibility is to the public. Those in government are chosen by the people and are responsible to them. Part of the responsibility of government in a democracy is to govern for the common good.	Capitalism is an economic system and has no interest in the common good or in public welfare. Corporations are required by law to serve the interests of their stockholders rather than the public good.
A democracy depends on people having access to information from multiple sources to make informed decisions, and there is public oversight into the finances and operations of the government.	Corporations are private entities and subject to no public oversight; they do not have to open their books or explain their actions.
Democracy is organized around government representing the interests of the people and is designed to protect and enforce protections against those who would harm the public good.	Governance is an entirely internal affair and the public has no input, no involvement.
Freedom of the Press is essential for the public to have access to full debate and contrasting views.	Capitalism as an economic system wants virtually no government interference, and insists that business be allowed to operate freely, governed only by market forces.
The essence of a democracy is free and fair elections, with every citizen having an equal voice and an equal vote.	Corporations seek to wield outsized amounts of power through lobbying and contributions to candidates and parties.
The public well-being is paramount. "Of, by, and for the people."	Profit is paramount for stockholders and high-level executives.
1 citizen = 1 vote	1 super Pac or billionaire = control of legislation and legislators through campaign finance and lobbying efforts.

Source: Author.

The intersection of the political class with the executives of the largest corporations has led to policies that increasingly favor the interests of the very wealthy. One example of that is the tax cut of 2018, that awarded great wealth to the wealthiest corporations and individuals and raised the national deficit by more than one trillion dollars. Capitalists such as the Koch brothers, Robert Mercer, Sheldon Adelson, and other billionaires have contributed hundreds of millions of dollars trying to elect candidates that will further their business interests. The tax cut very much furthers their business interests and is the payoff for their investments in the campaigns of those running for "higher office."

Another example is to look at the U.S. policy towards energy and towards climate change. Fossil fuel corporations, such as Exxon Mobil, and BP (British Petroleum) have intentionally misled the public about climate change in order to maximize their profits.

> The world's largest fossil fuel companies—BP, Chevron, ConocoPhillips, ExxonMobil, coal giant Peabody Energy, and Shell—were fully aware of the reality of climate change but continued to spend tens of millions of dollars to sow doubt and promote contrarian arguments they knew to be wrong. Taken together, the documents show that these six companies, in conjunction with the American Petroleum Institute (API)—the oil and gas industry's premier trade association—and a host of front groups, have colluded to intentionally deceive the public … (Negin, 2015)

The government has not only allowed this behavior to go on but has adopted energy policies that have rewarded the fossil fuel corporations, leading to immense profits. The current administration totally rejects scientific findings about climate change, has forbidden its scientists from speaking about the issue, has in some cases prohibited using the term "climate change" and has scrubbed its website clean of information that contradicts their insistence that there is no such thing as climate change.

Paul Buchheit, writing in 2013, called unregulated capitalism a cancer that was destroying the essence of U.S. society in its quest for ever expanding profits.

> The uncontrolled growth of investment wealth is diverting resources away from vital programs, effectively smothering them. […] Under capitalism, fortunes accrue to a few while 47 million Americans, or one out of seven, need food assistance. Almost half of the hungry are children. For every food bank we had in 1980, we now have 200. (Buchheit, 2013)

Buchheit says that "capitalism has betrayed our children [...] Child poverty, perhaps the main cause of their health problems, is up 50 percent since 1973, with the rate for minorities three times that for white children."

The Impact of U.S. Capitalism, Racism, and White Supremacy on the Larger World

I want to add a brief note into the discussion about the intersection of capitalism, racism, and white supremacy, and its impact on the health of people in this country and around the world. What capitalism has emphasized is "looking out for number one,"; it is all about "me," and winning at all costs no matter what the impact on anyone else.

Capitalism rewards self-centered behavior and applauds whatever individuals and corporations do to maximize profits and returns for their investors. This has led individuals and corporations to exploit the people, the land, the law, and whatever else in pursuit of those profits, and has led them to oppose those laws and protections that are geared toward the common good, the environment, and accountability for the actions taken.

Capitalism and white supremacy have justified the taking of lands occupied by indigenous people around the world, by any and every means necessary, and in what is now the United States, justified the policy of expanding and civilizing the "west," by driving out or murdering native populations living in those areas. They justified wars against native people and forced native people from their homes in the southeast in a forced migration to Oklahoma that led to the death of thousands (the Trail of Tears), so that whites could claim their former lands.

Ibram Kendi talks about the invention of racism and discriminatory policy as a way to justify and enable this exploitation that led those white men to enrich themselves and maintain their status at the top of their created hierarchy. Kendi says that discriminatory policy was

> [...] sprung from economic, political, and cultural self-interests. [...] Politicians seeking higher office have primarily created and defended discriminatory policies out of political self-interest—not racist ideas. Capitalists seeking to increase profit margins have primarily created and defended discriminatory policies out of economic self-interest—not racist ideas. Cultural professionals, including theologians, artists, scholars, and journalists, were seeking to advance their careers or cultures and have primarily created and defended discriminatory policies out of professional self-interest—not racist ideas [...] The beneficiaries of slavery, segregation, and mass

> incarceration have produced racist ideas of Black people being best suited for or deserving of the confines of slavery, segregation, or the jail cell. Consumers of these racist ideas have been led to believe there is something wrong with Black people, and not the policies that have enslaved, oppressed, and confined so many Black people. (Kendi, 2016, 10–11)

The policies of capitalism have led to the U.S. reaching beyond its borders to colonize and loot countries around the world. U.S. policy around the world was summed up succinctly by a sign carried during the protest march in Seattle on the eve of the Iraq invasion in 2003: "What is our oil doing under their sand?" The reach of U.S. corporations has exploited the populations, land, and resources of many countries, and has led to policies that have included invasion, launching more than fifty attempts at overthrowing governments since World War II (Blum, n.d.), wars in Korea, Vietnam, Iraq, Afghanistan, and elsewhere. The United States currently has more than eight hundred military bases in operation around the world, in over 80 countries, with an overall pentagon budget of more than 700 billion dollars annually.

Our current president's statement about "shithole countries," referring to many of the countries that the U.S. has exploited, his policies targeting Muslims and justifying the closing of American borders is about furthering the dominance of capitalism and the white race against a world that is increasingly non- white.

Seeing the Connections and Taking Action

The increasing inequality that we see in the United States (and around the world) is a consequence of these contradictory systems, the tension between serving the needs and interests of capital and serving the needs of the people, with the balance swinging strongly towards the dominating wealth of the upper one percent. In 2015, the average net worth of a member of Congress was more than one million dollars. Twenty percent of African American households have zero or negative net worth. Congress is making policies that widen the gap between the rich and the poor, and the idea that we are in this together is less and less true.

Can we have democracy and corporate capitalism? Can we have a democracy in a country that does not believe that Black lives matter? Or that Native American, or Latinx lives matter? Can we care about the health and well-being of all our people while corporations are legally bound to bring home as much to their investors as possible, no matter what the cost to the population or to the environment? Much depends on the resolution of that tension, that contradiction. And much depends on us recognizing that the seemingly isolated struggles we engage with day to day are like those isolated clumps of honey mushrooms, all part of an immense, underground organism that must finally be addressed if we are to make lasting change.

Challenging the extremes, the excesses of corporate capitalism and working to restore a greater balance between the needs of business and the needs of the public, working for the common good is obviously an overwhelming task when considered as a complete picture. How do we take on the Dark Money behind the curtains pulling the strings? They have the resources, they are in the power positions, they have the media, and they have little incentive to listen to us. What can we do?

My response, and what I will explore through the rest of the book is to keep our awareness on the big picture, on the underlying determinants of health that must be addressed at the policy level, but at the same time to focus on local actions, in our schools and in our communities. Local actions will help our children and our community in the short run and will also help us to build organization and momentum for larger actions. It will take time, longer than we want it to take and there will not be steady progress, but change can and will happen if we work together and stay focused on what matters most; the health and well-being of our children and neighbors, and of our planet.

The conservative, capitalist crowd worked for decades to engineer the changes we are now struggling with, and have been successful in doing so, sadly for the people and the planet, but it does mean that things can change, and will change if we organize and act.

One of the most effective places to start is within our schools, and that's what I will explore next.

References

Blum, W. (n.d.). Overthrowing other people's governments: The master list. Retrieved from https://williamblum.org/essays/read/overthrowing-other-peoples-governments-the-master-list

Buchheit, P. (2013). 5 ways that raw, unregulated capitalism is acting like a cancer on American society. Alternet. Retrieved from https://www.alternet.org/economy/5-ways-raw-unregulated-capitalism-cting-cancer-american-society?page=0,1&akid=10422.1125860.WPUmaz&rd=1&src=newsletter838402&t=19

Bush, G. W. (2001, July 4). Remarks by the President in Independence Day Celebration, Independence Historic National Park, Philadelphia, Pennsylvania. Retrieved from https://georgewbush-whitehouse.archives.gov/news/releases/2001/07/text/20010704-2.html

Chomsky. (2004). In Noam Chomsky: Language and politics, 2nd edition. (Otero, C. P., editor). New York: AK Press.

Civiced.org. (n.d.). The concepts and fundamental principles of Democracy. Retrieved from http://www.civiced.org/pdfs/books/ElementsOfDemocracy/Elements_Subsection3.pdf

Douglass, F. (1852.). What, to the slave is the 4th of July? Freeman Institute. Retrieved from http://www.freemaninstitute.com/douglass.htm

Fleming, N. (2014, November 19). The largest living thing on earth is a humongous fungus. BBC: Earth. Retrieved from http://www.bbc.com/earth/story/20141114-the-biggest-organism-in-the-world

Kasser, T. & Linn, S. (2016, January). Growing Up under Corporate Capitalism: The Problem of Marketing to Children, with Suggestions for Policy Solutions. Social Issues & Policy Review. Vol. 10 Issue 1, pp. 122–150. Retrieved from http://resolver.ebscohost.com.webdb.plattsburgh.edu:2048/openurl?sid=google&auinit=T&aulast=Kasser&atitle=Growing+up+under+corporate+capitalism%3a+The+problem+of+marketing+to+children%2c+with+suggestions+for+policy+solutions&id=doi%3a10.1111%2fsipr.12020&title=Social+Issues+%26+Policy+Review&volume=10&issue=1&date=2016&spage=122&site=ftf-live

Kendi, I. (2016). Stamped from the beginning. New York: Nation Books.

Kraus, M. W., & Tan, J. J. X. (2015, May). Americans overestimate social class mobility. Journal of Experimental Social Psychology,Volume 58, Pages 101–111. Retrieved from https://www.sciencedirect.com/science/article/pii/S0022103115000062#

Monaghan, A. (2014, November 13). U.S. wealth inequality—top 0.1% worth as much as the bottom 90%. The Guardian. Retrieved from https://www.theguardian.com/business/2014/nov/13/us-wealth-inequality-top-01-worth-as-much-as-the-bottom-90

Negin, E. (2015). Internal documents show fossil fuel industry has been aware of climate change for decades. Huffington Post. Retrieved from https://www.huffingtonpost.com/elliott-negin/internal-documents-show-f_b_7749988.html

· 6 ·

THE PURPOSE OF EDUCATION

I ask each group of new teacher candidates three connected questions: Why do we have school, what should happen at school, and who should decide what is taught at school? The students look at each other in some confusion; it is not a question they have really considered before. Their first responses are what you might expect. We go to school because it's what you do, because it's what we've always done, or that we need to go to school so we can learn what we need to learn so we can be successful adults. And we study what they tell us to study. There are requirements. It does not occur to them to ask why there are those requirements, who made those decisions, or to ask if there is something that could be more useful to them. It's what you do.

There is clearly more to this story, and the purpose and function of schools remains a question. There are deep struggles over curriculum, particularly in social studies, reading, and science, and deeper struggles over who should decide what is taught in those subjects. Some districts have made decisions in recent years to whitewash or eliminate what they deem to be uncomfortable history. Some states have changed the order things are taught in, or the year in which certain curriculum is introduced in response to testing. Some schools require everyone to teach the same thing at the same time; others give teachers room to make teaching decisions based on their sense of what will best serve the students.

In some ways schools look the way they have looked for hundreds of years, and in other ways they have changed dramatically from the time that many of us attended them, a few years or decades ago. The questions I want to explore in this chapter center around the fundamental question of what should schools be doing, who should decide that question, and on what basis should those decisions be made? These are not just theoretical questions. Consider what is happening in Michigan and Texas.

Michigan has just proposed changes in their social studies curriculum that

> [...] cuts out references to gay rights, Roe v. Wade and climate change. It also slashes the word "democratic" and replaces it with "republic." Behind the draft is Republican State Senator and Gubernatorial candidate Patrick Colbeck. He said his suggestions were motivated by concern that some standards are not politically neutral or factually accurate, and to ensure students are exposed to multiple points of view [...] (Strachan, 2018)

In 2010, Texas had its own curriculum revisions.

> Among other things, the revisions in Texas raised questions about the separation of church and state and determined that the inaugural address of the president of the Confederacy, Jefferson Davis, should be studied alongside Abraham Lincoln's. The word "capitalism," which some board members felt had negative connotations, was replaced with "free enterprise system."
>
> Cynthia Dunbar, a Republican board member from Richmond, set the tone for Friday's meeting when she opened it with an invocation.
>
> "I believe no one can read the history of our country without realizing that the Good Book and the spirit of the Savior have from the beginning been our guiding geniuses," she said.
>
> Conservatives on the board said the changes restore balance to a curriculum that has been tilted to the left after years of Democratic dominance on the board. Last year, the board approved changes in science-curriculum standards so that they now raise questions about evolution and global warming. Those changes provoked a similar outcry from college professors nationwide. (Mangan, 2010)

And in Texas again, this time in 2015:

> The Texas board of education adopted a revised social studies curriculum in 2010 after a fierce battle. When it came to social studies standards, conservatives championing causes from a focus on the biblical underpinnings of our legal system to a whitewashed picture of race in the United States won out. The guidelines for teaching Civil War history were particularly concerning: They teach that "sectionalism, states' rights and slavery"—carefully ordered to stress the first two and shrug off the

> last—caused the conflict. Come August, the first textbooks catering to the changed curriculum will make their way to Texas classrooms.
>
> It is alarming that 150 years after the Civil War's end children are learning that slavery was, as one Texas board of education member put it in 2010, "a side issue." No serious scholar agrees. (Washington Post, 2015)

Now more than ever it is crucial to recognize that public education is not neutral, and that what is in textbooks is not neutral, that public education is contested territory, and that the decisions made have an impact on the health and well-being of our students. When Howard Zinn wrote his memoir, *You Can't Be Neutral on a Moving Train* he was, among other things making the case that there is no such thing as a neutral, unbiased education. He challenged the argument that teachers should simply teach the curriculum the state hands them, because that's unbiased, and they should simply use the texts they are given, because they are unbiased. There is no such thing as unbiased, and the decisions about what is taught and how it is taught reflects the knowledge, beliefs, and values of whoever is making the decisions.

I have interviewed many potential teacher candidates in my role as a professor in teacher education programs and one of my first questions has been, why do you want to teach? The responses to that question have remained relatively constant through the years; the incoming students are still bright, caring young people who are pursuing teaching because they want to help younger people, to make a difference, as was true for those coming before them.

But something has changed in recent years to the next set of questions I ask, about what they want students they work with to get from being in their future classrooms. They are less sure, less willing to lay out their vision for what they hope will happen than were students who came before them. What has changed, what is different is that students coming into college in recent years have had their entire K-12 experience under No Child Left Behind. Students coming to college have been taught to be much more passive, obedient, and reluctant to take initiative when it comes to their own learning, so they come with more doubts and less confidence. They have been trained to follow the teacher's directions, all geared toward passing tests, and it does not occur to them that they can make different choices. They want to help their future students to be successful, which now means doing what they are told to do by their administrators, and mostly involves doing what is necessary to pass the standardized tests. Why are they doing that? Because that's what they were told to do. Beyond that, there is little clarity about what their education means or what it should or could mean. Considering what is going on in places like Texas and Michigan, that is a troubling attitude to carry into a classroom.

The Purpose of Education and the Role That Schools Play Within That

Societies educate their young; it's what they do to maintain their existence and to offer their children their best chance of surviving and flourishing. This education comes through many channels: through observation, from being with family, through working on the family farm or in the family business, through apprenticeships or mentorships or a series of jobs, through involvement in various organizations and groups, through going off to study, through living day to day. Some learning comes through religious institutions, some through other formal settings, through one to one encounters with adults, and some through individual journeys and meditations. Some of what we learn helps us to grow and expand our world, and unfortunately some of what we learn keeps our world somewhat constricted and closed.

When I think of my own education it has come from that same wide range of sources, and only a small portion of my fundamental education came from school. Much more came from family, friends, and the neighborhood in which I grew up. Part of that learning, I only realized later, reinforced some aspects of racism and privilege that I've spent much of my life working to unlearn, or to move beyond, and that work continues.

My learning continued with moves farther out into the world, first to Philadelphia and then to the Adirondack Mountains, to environments and contexts that put me in new situations with very different populations than I had known, with activism and experience while at college, with the challenges of independent living as a young adult. And I've continued to learn, through a long career, through a long marriage and parenting, and now grandparenting, and through the experiences, relationships, and challenges that come from living in the world.

I was also educated (and mis-educated) by the media, including television, which was a new, black and white three-channel presence in our household. We watched those few sports events that were televised, saw a heavy dose of westerns glorifying cowboys in their fight against "savage" Indians (played by non-Indian actors), part of the indoctrination that helped me to become mis-educated. I remember watching Walt Disney on Sunday evenings, with Davy Crockett, Indian fighter, helping to civilize the frontier, and later at the

Alamo, a hero fighting and dying at the hands of no-good Mexicans., There were many other shows featuring a cowboy hero standing for truth, justice, and the American way. Years later, as I learned of the genocide carried out by European "settlers" against Native Americans, and the land grab that was the "Mexican War," I realized more fully how Disney and those other programs had mis-educated me and millions of other viewers, about Davy Crockett, about the Civil War, about the interactions between European Americans and Native Americans, about gender roles, about race, and much else. Media played a major role for many of us in shaping how we viewed and (mis) understood the world, and it still does.

Schools Are Not the Same Thing as Education

We often talk about schools and education as if they were one and the same, and as I just shared, we learn through many different sources and in many different contexts. Some contexts and lessons prove particularly useful and relevant and they tend to stay with us; others not so much. Some of the most significant teachers I have found in my life have been in a school setting, but most have not. This is not a judgment on schools, but a realistic look at the learning I've done and where I've found it.

It's also important to keep in mind that there are many ways to "do" school; we tend to assume that all schooling resembles our own, which is far from the truth. Schools vary in size from very small, with graduating classes as small as ten, to schools serving thousands of students. Schools vary in the subjects they offer, the students they serve, the philosophies that guide their curricular and structural choices, the people who serve as teachers, and the ways the students are assessed. Many of the choices that have been made in how to design and run public schools in the U.S. were made more than a hundred years ago, in response to a society that in many ways does not resemble or respond to the world in which we now live.

I am not arguing against schooling; I have spent more than five decades in classrooms, as student and teacher, and highly value much of the experience, but I am also aware that schools are institutions created by and funded by the state, and like anything created by and funded by those in power, they serve the purposes of the state. In some cases that also serves the health and well-being of the students, but in too many cases it appears to do more harm than good to many of the students they purport to serve.

A Brief History of Schools

Schools have served many different functions throughout our history. They have answered to (and continue to answer to) multiple masters and have often worked at cross purposes in those conflicting roles. They have served individual students and communities by providing a relatively safe place for children to come together with caring adults to learn basic skills, to gain knowledge and awareness of the wider world, and to have access to possibilities broader than they might have found on their own. The early schools were gathering places for communities, often serving as the location for town meetings, social events, religious services, and governmental functions as well as the place where children came to learn some basic reading, writing, and arithmetic.

Schools have helped new immigrants to learn how to become Americans, have served as social service agencies supporting families by providing food, clothing, resources, basic medical care and connections to resources in the community. And they have opened some doors to potential employment, the arts, athletics, and relationships with the commons, providing a place for the community to come together.

Schools have been the place where we have learned the basic skills that society has decided we need to contribute to the common good, including basic reading and writing, some basic math, and a smattering of science, social studies, physical education. And it's the place where some of us have connected with an adult, a mentor who inspired a passion for a field, a topic, a question that launched us into our next years.

At the same time public schools have served to socialize young people towards unquestioning patriotism, towards automatic obedience to adults, and to a relatively narrow sense of possibilities. They have championed the role that America has played as a beacon of democracy and freedom while minimizing the full spectrum of costs and consequences that America's pursuit of wealth and power has brought to people here and around the world, and schools have taught us that our role was to fit in to society, to help maintain the status quo.

Who are schools for, who do they serve, and what should they offer? I want to offer a range of voices weighing in on these questions, perspectives that challenge the current and "traditional" approach to schooling that is hurting so many children, recognizing that there is not one right answer. My hope is that this range of voices stimulates and reminds us that education does not have to look like what we experienced. It does not have to take place in large buildings. It does not have to be structured so that all classes are the same size, last for the same number of minutes, no matter what is being taught, and are ruled by the same set of guidelines. Education can't and shouldn't be standardized, especially given the many different opinions of its purpose and how it should be carried out. And, most importantly, the purpose of education is not a settled question, but rather a question we have been forgetting to ask.

Here are the thoughts of a few thinkers to get the discussion started.

> The function of education is to teach one to think intensively and to think critically. But education which stops with efficiency may prove the greatest menace to society. The most dangerous criminal may be the man gifted with reason but no morals. [...] We must remember that intelligence is not enough. Intelligence plus character—that is the goal of true education. —Martin Luther King Jr., speech at Morehouse College, 1948

> Education is not the filling of a pail, but the lighting of a fire. —William Butler Yeats

> It seems to me that the role of educated beings is to suggest alternative frameworks, to imagine better ways of living and evolving worlds, to imagine new human relations that are free from persisting hierarchies, whether they be economic, racial, sexual, political. This is the spiritual significance of education. That significance is that education, critical education is truly the practice of freedom. Freedom then is not so much a state for which one yearns, but rather an incessant struggle to remake our lives, our relations, our communities, our democratic future. —Angela Davis

> Ideally, what should be said to every child, repeatedly, throughout his or her school life is something like this: 'You are in the process of being indoctrinated. We have not yet evolved a system of education that is not a system of indoctrination. We are sorry, but it is the best we can do. What you are being taught here is an amalgam of current prejudice and the choices of this particular culture. The slightest look at history will show how impermanent these must be. You are being taught by people who have been able to accommodate themselves to a regime of thought laid down by their predecessors. It is a self-perpetuating system. Those of you who are more robust and individual than others will be encouraged to leave and find ways of educating yourself—educating your own judgements. Those that stay must remember, always, and all the time, that they are being molded and patterned to fit into the narrow and particular needs of this particular society. —Doris Lessing, The Golden Notebook

> The whole educational and professional training system is a very elaborate filter, which just weeds out people who are too independent, and who think for themselves, and who don't know how to be submissive, and so on—because they're dysfunctional to the institutions. —Noam Chomsky

> We need to talk more about school as a place where young people form connections beyond the family to adults who can guide and mentor them [...] We need to talk

about school not only as a place where young people acquire knowledge, but where they learn how to use it, how to make an argument with historical events, how to think with numbers [...] We need to talk about self-reflection, becoming methodical, examining your own work. And we need to talk about reflecting on motive and on the consequences of choosing one path rather than another–whether in a science experiment or in the schoolyard [...] And all the above help young people develop a sense of themselves as knowledgeable and capable of acting in the world. This, finally, was what education gave me, a pathway from hazy disaffection to competence, to a dawning awareness that I could figure things out and do something with what I learned. This was the best training I could have gotten for vocation and citizenship. —Mike Rose

"School is the advertising agency which makes you believe that you need the society as it is." —Ivan Illich

Our care of the child should be governed, not by the desire to make him learn things, but by the endeavor always to keep burning within him that light which is called intelligence. —Maria Montessori

The purpose of school, I think, is three-fold. Ultimately, it's personal. It's about helping people find their personal talents, their abilities, and helping them become who they can be. Second, it's cultural. Education is also about helping people to understand the world they are part of. The background, the history, their own community and other people's communities, and the fact that they are part of a broader world that goes beyond them. And third is economic, it's helping people develop the skills and attitudes that will help them to make a living and contribute to the common good, the common welfare. [...] It's those three things, and if we lose sight of them we lose sight of education. —Sir Ken Robinson

The best sort of schooling is organized around problems, projects, and questions—as opposed to facts, skills, and disciplines. Knowledge is acquired, of course, but in a context and for a purpose. The emphasis is not only on depth rather than breadth, but also on discovering ideas rather than on covering a prescribed curriculum. —Alfie Kohn

The paradox of education is precisely this—that as one begins to become conscious one begins to examine the society in which he is being educated. The purpose of education, finally, is to create in a person the ability to look at the world for himself, to make his own decisions, to say to himself this is black or this is white, to decide for himself whether there is a God in heaven or not. To ask questions of the universe, and then learn to live with those questions, is the way he achieves his own identity. But no society is really anxious to have that kind of person around. What societies really, ideally, want is a citizenry which will simply obey the rules of society. If a society succeeds in this, that society is about to perish. The obligation of anyone who thinks of himself as responsible is to examine society and try to change it and to fight it—at no matter what risk. This is the only hope society has. This is the only way societies change. —James Baldwin, 1963

James Baldwin laid out the contradiction so clearly in his talk to teachers in 1963. What we want for our children, to be critical thinkers and passionate learners who care about others and who stand up for justice is someone that "no society is really anxious to have … around." That's it, in a nutshell. People who think for themselves, who can see through the smoke screens that politicians and governments and media outlets and history textbooks produce, to see the "men behind the curtain" are much more difficult to control, to program, and are more likely to challenge the injustice that serves those in power at the expense of those most distant from power. We may want it for our own children, but the thought of everyone's children thinking for themselves and acting in their own interests, and in the interests of communities that are not ours, seems to be perceived as a danger, a threat. It might produce "an excess of democracy."

An Excess of Democracy

When schools were more student centered during the 1960s and 1970s, and there were intentional efforts to connect what students were learning in the classroom to what was happening around them, students were taking their studies of democracy and movements for justice to the streets with demonstrations against the Vietnam War, demonstrations for Civil Rights, and demonstrations for women's rights. The Trilateral Commission, made up in part by people who would later become part of the Carter administration issued a report entitled "The Crisis of Democracy." The report cautioned against what they termed "an excess of democracy;" it said that "The effective operation of a democratic political system usually requires some measure of apathy and noninvolvement on the part of some individuals and groups" (Chomsky, 1981).

Samuel Huntington, one of the authors of the report, expressed his concern that this excess of democracy was bad for the country because it made the country look bad on the world stage. It was harder to be the leader around the world if it could not keep its own population in line. Huntington lamented the increasing actions and influence of the common people. He said,

"Truman had been able to govern the country with the cooperation of a relatively small number of Wall Street lawyers and bankers," but activism made this much more difficult by the mid-1960s. The population was much less governable because they were less willing to be submissive. Huntington notes that "previously passive or unorganized groups in the population," such as "blacks, Indians, Chicanos, white ethnic groups, students and women—all of whom became organized and mobilized in new ways to achieve what they considered to be their appropriate share of the action and of the rewards" were a threat to the smooth functioning of our democracy, which depended on "some measure of apathy and noninvolvement on the part of some individuals and groups" (Chomsky, 1981).

Chomsky's commentary echoes Baldwin's comments, that a well-educated population that knows its rights, knows the laws, and is able to think critically, to communicate effectively, to organize, and to act is a problem for leaders who want to simply issue orders that a population passively follows.

This contradiction places public education squarely in the center of the conflict between corporate capitalism and democracy, a tension I discussed briefly in the previous chapter. If we teach people to think for themselves, to think critically and to analyze the world around them and they find it unjust, they just might take what they feel are responsible actions to make it more just, challenging the status quo, which might be identified by the government as a danger, a threat. Having too much democracy in a democracy is a curious paradox, and one that really gets to the heart of the questions in this book. When the democracy stops being democratic, when the society based on serving the common good stops serving that common good, what does "right action" look like? Are schools doing their jobs when they educate people to notice the injustices and feel moved to act, using the skills and knowledge they gained from public education? The authors of the Trilateral Commission did not think so, and scolded institutions such as schools, churches and synagogues for failing to keep their populations passive.

The dictates coming down from the federal government and state governments are very much in line with this corporate capitalist agenda, emphasizing competition, with a focus on high stakes testing that rewards a few and punishes the rest, and which tolerates no excuses or activism. Schools across the country are tying themselves in knots trying to meet the high stakes testing mandates demanded by the federal and state governments with fewer and fewer resources, as what were once education dollars are diverted to the military and other business-related enterprises. It is a no-win for the schools, and as the funding fails and the demands rise the education of children is compromised. Each district is approaching its own financial disaster in isolation even though the districts right next door are experiencing similar struggles, and for the same underlying reasons. The state claims it can't fully fund education (no matter what state we're talking about) even as the costs for everything from transportation to electricity continue to rise.

It is a fundamental question that faces those of us in education, but it is essentially the same question that faces anyone working to support the health and well-being of the general population, and particularly those working with under-represented populations. We are losing local control, we are losing funding, we are losing the ability to adequately serve the most vulnerable populations, and as a consequence we are getting less healthy and whole as a people, and as a democracy. We have a choice to make; do we support the policies and institutions that are at the heart of democracy or do we continue down the current road we are on, where the drive for concentrated power and wealth in the hands of a few takes precedence over a focus on the common good? It seems clear that we can't serve both masters.

Education for Freedom or Conformity

For Brazilian educator Paulo Freire, the role of education is central in the reproduction of capitalist social relations.

> Education either functions as an instrument that is used to facilitate the integration of generations into the logic of the present system and bring about conformity to it, or it becomes the 'practice of freedom,' the means by which men and women deal critically with reality and discover how to participate in the transformation of their world. (Freire, 2000)

Freire's well-known banking theory says that

> Education thus becomes an act of depositing, in which the students are the depositories and the teacher is the depositor ... This is the banking concept of education, in which the scope of action allowed to the students extends only as far as receiving, filing, and storing the deposits. (Freire 1972, 58)

Freire saw this banking approach taken by the schools as no accident. "The capability of banking education to minimize or annul the students' creative power and to stimulate their credulity serves the interests of the oppressors, who care neither to have the world revealed nor to see it transformed" (Freire, 1972, 60).

He advocated instead for a liberatory approach to education. "Those truly committed to liberation must reject the banking concept in its entirety … They must abandon the educational goal of deposit-making and replace it with the posing of the problems of men (sic) in their relationship with the world" (Freire, 1972, 66).

Noam Chomsky also believes that are two basic views or models of what education should be, what he calls an enlightenment view and the indoctrination view.

Chomsky labels his own view as the enlightenment view, in which the

> […] highest goal in life is to inquire and create. The purpose of education from that point of view is just to help people to learn on their own. It's you the learner who is going to achieve in the course of education and it's really up to you to determine how you're going to master and use it. An essential part of this kind of education is fostering the impulse to challenge authority, think critically, and create alternatives to well-worn models. (Jones, 2012)

Chomsky defines the opposing concept of education as indoctrination. Under this model, "People have the idea that, from childhood, young people have to be placed into a framework where they're going to follow orders. This is often quite explicit." (Jones, 2012).

Millions of students are harmed by their K-12 experience. Many of the students I worked with at university had been taught to be afraid and to be compliant and these are students who were successful enough to make it to college and to be on the path to teaching. If this is what happens for the "successful" students, what is the story of those who don't succeed? Sadly, we know that story all too well: more than one million students drop out of high school every year (approximately seven thousand per day) and more than eighty percent of those in prison dropped out or were pushed out of high school. The harm done to them, to their families, to their communities can be measured in dollars, but there is a deeper and more fundamental damage done to families and communities that have lost their young men and women to prison, to drugs, to death. This is a major health issue, part of the social determinants that impact population health.

Which brings me back to the question of why schools? Who do they serve, who benefits and what do we want from them?

Educators have been wrestling with the question about the purpose of schools and seem to recognize that a choice has to be made between either meeting the needs of the students or meeting the needs of the state as a first priority. It can't do both.

What Is the Purpose of School?

Magdalena Slapik spoke with students about what they thought education was/should be; here are excerpts from two responses she published. The italics are in the original.

> *What do you think is the purpose of education, and what role should school play in a student's life?*
>
> *What is the role school and teachers should play in students' lives?*
>
> The role of education and the role of teachers is to empower students not just to do what they want, but to make mistakes. The more often you make mistakes, the more likely you will be to do something important. Messing up is something that we have to foster. Because, that's how expressing yourself works—it's when you get the chance to be wrong and to just sort of have a go at random things.
>
> That's the problem with our education system now [...] mistakes are the worst things you can make. The reason that that's bad is because it encourages students—when they take a test or when they study for something or when they do projects—to be dead inside. To sort of be sterilized. And music and the arts are about being fully alive, and about just being completely in the moment, where all your senses are enlivened and working. That's the kind of experience that school should foster and harness and be focused on. Not in trying to get everyone to line up and just sort of follow the rules and take orders. That kind of environment is really destructive.
>
> Emilia Olson, Grade 11
> Palmetto Scholars Academy—North Charleston, South Carolina
> (Magdalena Slapik / *The Hechinger Report*)
>
> *What role should school and teachers play in students' lives?*
>
> When a student goes to a certain school, they all come from different backgrounds, different upbringings: who was home, who took care of them, how much they saw them, what their occupation was. All these factors make them all different. I feel like school should be a place where I can learn about their culture and where they came from and them learn about mine. And, of course, you know, have your science and math, and learn how to write. But also be, not necessarily a culture shock, but a place to broaden your mind.
>
> If you don't do it young, then you'll never do it, in my opinion. If we don't start appreciating the kid next to you who has a completely different family style or family structure and life experience, then you won't do it when you're older. You'll look at it in a single-track way. I feel like that's the role of a teacher and school as an institution. Just to create a space where students can fail, and still be like, "OK, I'm gonna try again, but in a different way." Instead of saying, "Ok, I failed. I'm not going to be anything. Let me just quit." Ifetayo Kitwala, Grade 11

The young people echo both Freire and Chomsky but in their own words. The role of education is to help students to stay alive, to learn by doing, with support, to find their own truths through trial and error, through making mistakes, through meeting and learning with others who are different, who have different experiences and ways of making meaning in the world. They are advocating a school experience that is anything but standardized, rote learning.

Schools and the Status Quo

One response to that question of "why schools?" comes from Rich Gibson, emeritus professor from San Diego State University and co-founder of the Rouge Forum, an organization of educators, historians, and activists committed to challenging the status quo and working for equity and justice. Gibson has written about a workshop he has presented at conferences entitled "Why School?" In the workshop he raises the initial question and, based on the responses he gets moves the conversation on to other questions such as these: What are the Key Things Happening in Schools Today? What are the Key Things Happening in Society? From This Analysis, What Shall We Do and Think?

Here is how he answers the question he poses to others:

> Schools are huge multi-billion-dollar markets where profit and loss always influence almost everything. Consider the busses, the architects, textbook sales, consultants, the developers for the buildings, the upkeep, the grounds, the sports teams, salaries, etc. Cost is always an issue in school. This is, after all, capitalism. [...] This answer can lead to other good interrogations like: Is there a single public school system in the U.S. (or wherever)? Actually, there is not. There are five or six carefully segregated school systems, based mostly on class and race. The capitalist market necessarily creates inequality, not only in the pocket, but in the mind.
>
> There is a pre-prison school system in Detroit or Compton, a pre-Walmart system in National City, a pre-craft worker system in City Heights, a pre-teacher or social worker system in Del Cero, a pre-med or pre-law system in La Jolla and Birmingham, and a completely private school system where rich people send their kids, like George W. Bush or Mitt Romney.
>
> Rich schools teach different realities using different methods from poor schools. In rich schools the outlook is: 'This globe is ours; let us see how we can make it act.' In the poorest schools, the outlook is, 'Tell me what to do and I will do it.' (Gibson, n.d.)

Schools have served to keep the status quo and to quell resistance to it. As the industrial revolution came into full swing, schools helped to industrialize the population, which included teaching basic skills and habits that would make adults more effective and compliant workers, but also helped to minimize conflicts between the rich and the poor. There was tremendous fear on the part of the wealthy that class conflict between labor and capital was a real danger, and they enlisted schools in their efforts to keep down the unruly masses. Historian David Tyack quotes an educator as saying, "If we were to define the public school as an instrument for disintegrating mobs, we would indicate one of its most important purposes" (Tyack, 1974, 74). Horace Mann, the so-called father of public education referred to lower classes as "wild beasts, that prove their right to devour by showing their teeth." It was Mann's hope that by bringing together children from diverse segments of the population to a common school he could tame the wild beast and forestall revolution or violent uprisings (Tyack, 1974).

Schools have served a society that has become more unequal over the past thirty or more years, and we have seen that inequality has threatened and worsened the health of our population.

And now the purpose of schools, the definition of being well educated has become performance on standardized tests. They are the only thing that matter. When I have asked people what they want for their children, and for other people's children from schools they have generated a consistent list, which I presented in chapter one; children who are creative, curious, resilient, kind, and so on.

That list is now irrelevant when it comes to evaluating schools, teachers, and the students themselves. It's all about passing those tests and the most curious thing is that the obsession with testing actually undermines education in support of what we say we want for our children. When students are being trained to take the tests, they are being trained away from developing their creativity, compassion, critical thinking, independence, and the other traits we say we value most highly.

Aligning Policies With Values

Schools and districts must decide where their priorities lie, to whom they owe their primary allegiance, and then align their policies with that allegiance. The public schools are financed by local funds (about forty four percent), by state funding (about forty five percent) and by federal dollars (about ten percent). There is enormous pressure to follow the dictates of the federal and state mandates, to standardize schools, to keep funding and to avoid punishments including possible state takeover. This means sticking with the program, standardizing the education that students receive and the assessment that determines if they have met expectations.

On the other hand, schools can choose to focus on that which produces and sustains health and well-being for students, which focuses on the physical, social, economic, spiritual, and academic/intellectual needs of the students. It helps them develop as whole beings, able to work alone and with others, to think critically, to work cooperatively, and to be supportive of and appreciative of the well-being of others.

Coming back to the range of quotes that began this chapter, there are a few that help me to crystalize the tensions surrounding the question. The four voices who are most positive and clear about the value of schools focus on how they can help individuals find their way. They bring the narrowest lens to thinking about education, focusing on how they can best serve the individual.

Schools were a life saver for Mike Rose. They gave him a place to find himself and the tools with which to do that. He sees school as a place where students can find each other, can find and work with mentors who support them to "develop a sense of themselves as knowledgeable and capable of acting in the world."

Ken Robinson finds in schools a three-fold purpose: personal, helping students to find their personal talents and abilities, to help them become who they can be; cultural, helping students to become aware of the world they are a part of; and economic, helping them to learn what they need to in order to support themselves economically.

William Butler Yeats sees education as the lighting of a fire, where an individual can become inspired and passionate about the world.

Maria Montessori also used fire and light as images for education. She saw the goal of education to keep the light of intelligence lit, to inspire individuals to stay alive to the world.

Alfie Kohn sees the purpose of schools as to help students learn how to learn, for a purpose. He sees them investigating questions that matter to them and going for depth, for real understanding rather than memorizing a "bunch o'facts," as he calls them. The payoff for this type of education is discovering ideas, in learning something new that leads to other new ideas and possibilities. He is focused on the individual, as are others who are more positive about the potential in schools, but he is opposed to schools as a kind of training for becoming a contestant on Jeopardy, which he sees in the current test centered approach.

The more critical voices focus less on the impact that schools have on individuals and more on the role that schools play in society. Schools for these three are geared towards maintaining the status quo, indoctrinating students into toeing the line and following the path that is set out for them and helping to maintain that status quo by filtering out those who don't fit, who will challenge or cause problems. The role of schools in their view is first to maintain and sustain society as it is, with the needs of the individual students of secondary importance.

Ivan Illich sees schools as selling the status quo and encouraging students not to question or challenge.

Noam Chomsky sees education as a filter that weeds out or discards those who "are too independent and who think for themselves and who don't know how to be submissive." They are too hard to deal with, too difficult for the system since they don't just go along with the program.

Novelist Doris Lessing was even harder on schools, calling them systems of indoctrination, "an amalgam of current prejudice and the choices of this particular culture," as she phrases it.

And there are three who offer both a sense of hope mixed with a strong sense of caution.

Dr. King, in an early speech offered a complex view, still focused on the individual. He recognized the value of schools "in teaching one to think intensively and to think critically," but cautioned the need to couple that with morality. He phrased it as "Intelligence plus character," and worried that someone who was gifted but with no morals could be an incredible danger to society.

James Baldwin perfectly captured the impossible contradiction that schools offer; a place to learn to think critically, to learn about the world and to understand how things fit together, and the realization that if you are too successful at learning these things you become a danger to society, a person no one wants around.

And finally, Angela Davis offers an aspirational lens to the role that education can play in serving the larger society, bridging the voices. She says the 'role of educated beings is to suggest alternative frameworks, to imagine better ways of living and evolving worlds. […] That education, critical education is truly the practice of freedom, which she further defines as "not so much a state for which one yearns, but rather an incessant struggle to remake our lives, our relations, our communities, our democratic future."

What Do We Value?

We know that societies educate their young so that their young have the best possible chance of surviving to a happy and healthy adulthood, to have children of their own so that the society itself survives and sustains. There is no single recipe for how that education happens, what it consists of, who makes decisions about it, or much else. What does seem clear is that the educational approach or system that a society chooses is a reflection of what they value. They educate those children they feel it is important to educate in a way that will prepare them to enter the society as it is, or how they want it to be. Education can't be viewed separately from the society in which it exists, which also means that it can't be changed or "fixed" without changing the underlying foundation upon which it rests.

Finland decided to change its educational system in the 1960s and moved from a mediocre system to one of the world's most respected systems. They decided that their most important resource was their people, and that a strong educational system was one of the most important investments they could make.

> One of the basic principles of Finnish education is that all people must have equal access to high-quality education and training. The same educational opportunities should be available to all citizens irrespective of their ethnic origin, age, wealth or where they live. (Finnish National Agency for Education, 2011)

Finland established as a national policy "to build a better pathway out of poverty and into a productive life" (Saunders, 2016). They decided to move towards a more equitable society and educational system so that students were receiving good food and a good education no matter where they were living, no matter where they were attending school. There is little difference in student performance from one school to the next in Finland, because they are essentially equivalent experiences. It is a choice they made at the societal, governmental level and took the steps necessary to make that change. It comes out of a philosophy that each person is important and deserves the best education possible so that they can contribute to a society that needs everyone contributing to be successful. Their educational choice aligns with their economic system, one based on a need for all to contribute, and a belief that there should not be wide gaps between those who have and those who lack.

The United States has alternated between a move towards a more inclusive, democratic society and a more rigid, competitive and restrictive society through much of its history as I shared in the previous chapter. During its more democratic swing in the 1960s and early 1970s the schools were more democratic and child centered, more like what Finland has moved towards in recent decades. There was much more attention paid to the social and emotional needs of children, there was a recognition that children learn differently, and that one approach does not serve everyone. There was more room for schools to explore different approaches to teaching and learning as educators looked for ways to reach and teach as many of their students as possible.

Since the later 1970s and on through present day the society has moved away from the democratic end of its pendulum swing and has moved towards the corporate capitalist/economic end of the pendulum. The schools have followed suit, becoming more competitive, more rigid, and less welcoming to those who learn differently and don't fit the mold. When No Child Left Behind passed congress in 2002, this reflected the philosophy of the corporate capitalist value system. NCLB is a system that values individualism, believes in winners and losers, and believes in standards and efficiency with no excuses. It is largely based on the eugenics theory that says there is a superior race and they deserve to have dominion over the other races. The high stakes testing requirements of NCLB, emphasizing scores on tests that are biased racially and economically, fulfill that function.

It is not a mystery nor a surprise that a society's education system aligns with the values of its decision makers, and so what we are seeing in the United States is an education system that fits the economic designs of its rulers. There is not one, equal public school system, as they have in Finland. Instead there are several systems at play, each serving a different role for a different population, as Rich Gibson makes clear in his essay/workshop "Why School?" cited a few pages back.

Gibson sees that the ruling class cares much more about educating its own children, preparing them to become the next generation of rulers than it does in offering an equal education to the children of others, who are educated so that they fit into the role they are slotted to fill, somewhere lower down in the hierarchy. The purpose of education in this model is to maintain the status quo, which maintains the ruling class at the top of the hierarchy.

The question that faces us, finally, as we confront the purpose of education, is inextricably tied to our deep questions about who we are as a country, as a people. We must decide whether we lean towards caring and sharing, using our resources and talents to work towards the common good, or towards a system that values a more individualistic, looking out for number one system that rewards competition and profits.

References

Baldwin, J. (1963). A talk to teachers. Retrieved from http://richgibson.com/talktoteachers.htm

Chomsky, N. (1981). The Carter administration: Myth and reality. Radical Priorities (excerpt). Retrieved from https://chomsky.info/priorities01/

Finnish national agency for education. (2011). Finnish education in a nutshell. Finnish Ministry of Education. Retrieved from https://www.oph.fi/download/146428_Finnish_Education_in_a_Nutshell.pdf

Freire, P. (2000). Pedagogy of the oppressed. London: Continuum Press, p. 34.

Freire, P. (1972). Pedagogy of the oppressed. New York: Herder and Herder, p. 58.

Gibson, R. (n.d.). March 4th: Why have school? Retrieved from http://richgibson.com/gibson.htm

Jones, K. (2012). What is the purpose of education? Retrieved from http://www.forbes.com/sites/sap/2012/08/15/what-is-the-purpose-of-education

Mangan, K. (2010, May 23). Ignoring experts' pleas, Texas board approves controversial curriculum standards. The Chronicle of Higher Education. Retrieved from https://www.chronicle.com/article/Texas-Board-Approves/65661

Saunders, D. (2016, April 22). Finland's social climbers: How they're fighting inequality with education, and winning. Globe 2 Go. Retrieved from https://www.theglobeandmail.com/news/national/education/how-finland-is-fighting-inequality-with-education-andwinning/article29716845/

Slapik, M. (2017, October 1). The purpose of education—according to students. The Atlantic. Retrieved from https://www.theatlantic.com/education/archive/2017/10/the-purpose-of-education-according-to-students/541602/

Strachan, J. (2018, June 21). Proposed social studies changes rewrite history, incite outcry. Detroit Patch. Retrieved from https://patch.com/michigan/detroit/proposed-social-studies-changes-rewrite-history-incite-outcry

Tyack, D. (1974). The one best system. Cambridge: Harvard Press, p. 74

Washington Post Editorial Board. (2015). How Texas is whitewashing Civil War history. Washington Post. Retrieved from https://www.washingtonpost.com/opinions/whitewashing-civil-war-history-for-young-minds/2015/07/06/1168226c-2415-11e5-b77f-eb13a215f593_story.html?utm_term=.3bc5889cf098

· 7 ·

HIGH-STAKES STANDARDIZED TESTING

I want to start this chapter on high-stakes testing by reviewing what people I've spoken with say they want for their children because it is important to hold that in front of us when we consider what is happening in the schools and the role that the testing is playing. They value children being creative, persistent, flexible, effective problem solvers and able to work with others. They want their children to be critical thinkers, people who care about others and who value the full spectrum of people they meet. They want their children to grow into people who will be responsible members of families, good husbands or wives or partners, good parents, good neighbors, active and responsible community members who will stand up for what they believe, and who will also listen to and consider the points of view of others. They want them to become successful adults. And most of all, they want their children to be happy and healthy, to grow up able to realize their potential. There is little disagreement about the items on the list, though we might have debates about how we would weight and value them in relation to each other.

Given the general agreement about what we want for our children it is both curious and troubling that we have as a society thrown this list over in terms of what is valued and required of our public schools. What matters now, and really the only thing that has come to matter in public schools, is student and school performance on standardized tests in ELA, math, and, in some cases, science.

That's it. Are they good classmates? Doesn't matter? Are they curious? It's probably easier if they aren't as there isn't time for their questions or interests; they have to get to World War II by … or the Vietnam War by … and then the Iraq War by … Are they resilient? They'd better be, because this is a no-excuses operation. High-stakes decisions are based on those test scores. New teachers are promoted or left behind based to a significant degree on the scores of their students. Curricula and curriculum materials are promoted, purchased (at great expense), or left behind based on whether they lead students to the test-centered promised land. Schools and districts are ranked based on those test scores and on whether they have been successful at bullying/cajoling/manipulating students and families to take the tests and to take them seriously.

While there is virtually no evidence and no research to show that this test-centric approach leads to a better education and future (and no agreement about what better education even looks like much less how to assess it), and while there is significant evidence to show that the tests are in fact harmful and stressful to many of the students, families, and educators they involve, there has been no serious consideration about rethinking this hyper-focus on testing. In fact, those who have dared to speak out against the policy have been disciplined (or threatened with discipline), transferred, or shut down in other ways.

This raises some obvious questions. Why are we as a nation currently wedded to the system as it is? Why are those in power so dismissive of evidence that contradicts the approach, so punitive against those who would challenge it and so committed to this questionable path?

High-stakes, standardized testing has become the center point of public education since the passage of No Child Left Behind in 2002 and has brought significant change to the nation's schools, and yet, even now, sixteen years later, most people really don't know much about the law or how schools have been changed by it. A little history might help to start the conversation.

How Did We Get Here?

Civil Rights legislation in the mid-1960s included the Elementary and Secondary Education Act (ESEA), a response to the warehousing of African-American children in newly integrated schools. The schools had been forced by the Supreme Court's Brown v. Board of Education decision of 1954 to integrate, but that did not require them to actually educate the African-American students they had been ordered to allow into their buildings. Instead, many schools would send the African-American students to classrooms in remote corners and essentially ignore them. ESEA sought to change that, requiring that schools teach all students and demonstrate that they were doing so through some sort of assessment practice. Congress was required to reauthorize the law every five years and did so without significant change up through 2002. That's when most everything changed.

No Child Left Behind, as the 2002 reauthorization came to be called, required that all students take standardized tests in ELA and math, and pass them. Schools and districts had to have a ninety-five percent pass rate in every demographic category by 2014 or face increasingly draconian punishment, each year worse than the previous one, culminating in state takeover or school closure. There was much rhetoric about how these tests would close the achievement gap between students of color and white students, and there were politicians such as Ted Kennedy who supported the move as a step towards racial and social justice. Schools in Houston had used this approach and supposedly had turned their schools around. People were calling it the "Texas Miracle," and George W. Bush brought the Houston superintendent to Washington D. C. to become his secretary of education. Bush said that what happened in Houston could happen across the county.

In an odd way Bush was prophetic. What had happened in Houston turned out to be a fraud; there was no Texas miracle, no dramatic turnaround in Houston schools, no closing of the gap between students of color and white students. And there has been no turnaround or miracles in schools around the country. The gap between test scores of students of color and white students has not closed, and the test scores of all students have stayed relatively flat. Despite the clear failure of NCLB, public education continues down the high stakes testing road, continuing to spend hundreds of millions of dollars and wasting hundreds of hours of teaching time and of children's lives preparing them to take high stakes tests that are worthless as assessment and that have introduced significant stress into school districts and classrooms.

There are so many problems with high-stakes standardized testing that it is hard to know where to begin, but I will share a few of the concerns about this testing policy.

There Is No Such Thing as a Standardized Child

The late educational policy researcher Gerald Bracey used to say that there is no such thing as a standardized test because there is no such thing as a standardized child. We are unique, with our own mix of traits, skills, challenges, and ways of moving through the world. While Bracey's observation can simply stand on its own, I will go into a bit more detail about how and why we are unique, and how attempts to standardize the educational system are deeply flawed and perhaps driven by motives other than a desire to improve public education.

There Is No Such Thing as a Standardized Neighborhood: Test Scores and Zip Codes

Students who live in wealthy neighborhoods score better on standardized tests, on average than do students who live in poorer neighborhoods. Research has shown that students living in communities of lower-income are more likely to: suffer from more stress in early childhood, have more limited access to enriching educational resources, and receive less exposure to spoken language and vocabulary early in life. Studies show that poverty can change the structure of the brain. Recent research concerning people living in poverty "suggests the limbic system is constantly sending fear and stress messages to the prefrontal cortex, which overloads its ability to solve problems, set goals, and complete tasks in the most efficient ways" (Mathewson, 2017).

Martin West, an associate professor at the Harvard Graduate School of Education, says that the income achievement gap continues to widen:

> The gap in student achievement, as measured by test scores between low-income and high-income students, is a pervasive and longstanding phenomenon in American education, and indeed in education systems around the world. (West quoted in Bergland, 2015)

In Chapter 2 I shared research from David Berliner (2009) in which he found that as much as sixty percent of what happens in schools is due to out-of-school factors, which includes family wealth and income. Families with relatively strong incomes are able to send their children to schools that are stable, well resourced, and staffed by veteran teachers. They have the latest educational materials, have families that can afford to take time to get involved, have libraries and school librarians, and a tax base to support their work.

Families living in low-income neighborhoods have fewer resources with which to support their schools. Many of the families are struggling to simply meet their day-to-day needs so there is more stress in the household. More of the children are bringing additional stress and health-related challenges to the school. While quality education can and does happen in schools serving low-income communities, there are more hurdles, and more challenges to face. Inequality of living conditions, inequality of resources and facilities, and inequality in the support that families can offer their children highlight the absurdity of pretending that there is such a thing as a standardized test that can honestly and accurately compare the performance of students and schools. Test scores are not a reflection of how smart the children are, however that is defined, nor of the quality or dedication of the teaching staff, nor a measure of the caring of the families.

There Is No One Assessment That Measures Intelligence

We each encounter the world differently; no two people have the same experience, even when engaged in similar behaviors. People living in rural Louisiana, San Francisco, or the middle of Montana live very different lives economically, socially, and academically, and what they are taught to value and learn is shaped by where they are and with whom.

I am a white, middle-class male living in a system that privileges white middle (and upper-class) males. I come from an intact family of readers. We went to museums and concerts and other cultural events. My family did crossword puzzles and math games at the kitchen table. My teachers looked like my parents. The tests were designed to assess people like me. I have had virtually every advantage I could have, and I'm only too aware of my good fortune, my privilege when I compare my life to the lives of some of my students, who have faced many more hurdles than I will ever know. And I'm painfully aware that much of my privilege has been at the expense of the communities from which many of my students come. The policy of high-stakes standardized testing is a cynical mythology, another example of a weaponized policy that justifies white supremacy and blames those who have been discriminated against for their "failures."

There Is No Such Thing as Standardized Development or Maturation

We know that children develop and mature on their own timelines, shaped by genetics; by family; by economics and social factors; by race, class, gender, and environment; by their encounters with educators, friends, and myriad other factors. Any attempt at forcing people into a standardized schedule of maturation or development violates and contradicts all we know about learning, and development. The idea of a standardized test at third grade, for example, is based on the flawed notion that all third graders should be at a certain point in their learning and development at the time they are taking the test. It reflects an industrial mode of thinking, that all widgets should move along the assembly line at the same pace and be ready for packing and shipping on the same date. But children are not widgets.

Intelligence Testing and Standardized Testing Are Based on Racist Theory From the Eugenics Movement

The notion that there is a way to use a single instrument that can produce a single score that accurately measures intelligence comes out of the eugenics movement, as I've already discussed. There is quite a bit of evidence that the tests are biased and that the consistent gap in test results have more to do with the biases of the tests and the out-of-school factors that I shared in chapter two than they do with the inherent intelligence or learning capabilities of any race or ethnicity (Au, 2009).

No Expert in Research Would Support Making High-Stakes Decisions on Taking a Single Test

There are no testing experts who would claim that it is valid to use one of their tests as the sole basis for making significant decisions, and yet that is how standardized tests are being used. Bob Howard and I found these instructions included in testing materials from Riverside Publishing, which produced the Washington Assessment of Student Learning, the standardized test then in use across Washington State:

> While school and district scores may be useful in curriculum and instructional planning it is important to exercise extreme caution when interpreting individual reports. [...] Scores from one test given on a single occasion should never be used to make important decisions about students' placement, the type of instruction they receive, or retention in a given grade level in school. [...] When making decisions about individuals, multiple sources of information should be used. Multiple individuals who are familiar with the student's progress and achievement—including parents, teachers,

> school counselors, school psychologists, specialist teachers, and perhaps the students themselves—should be brought together to collaboratively make such decisions. (Howard and Selwyn, 2008, 276)

The Tests Are Culturally Biased, Favoring Students With Certain Kinds of Experiences and Knowledge

I have already spoken about the classes of students I worked with who were second-language learners, who were relatively recent immigrants, and who struggled with the standardized tests. There is now extensive research showing how the tests are not only a struggle for readers and writers working in a second language but are culturally biased such that students who are not white and middle class are less likely to score well on the tests. In fact, there is research showing that questions that have African-American students scoring higher than white students are thrown out because they are not "performing" as they should (Rosner, 2003). There are issues of familiarity with the culture assumed by the questions, and the very format of the testing is more comfortable for certain students than it is for others. The consistent differential in test scores between members of certain races and classes at the very least calls into question the validity and reliability of the tests and should raise questions about whether these tests should be the basis for significant decisions.

Students With Special Needs Must Take the Tests

Students with special needs are required to take the tests, no matter how inappropriate it might be for them to do so. Students who have significant learning disabilities, who struggle in any number of ways are still expected to sit for several hours, along with their classmates engaging in what for them is an impossible and humiliating task. We have seen that requiring people to engage in tasks that they can't possibly succeed in and then judging them raises their stress levels significantly. In what ways does this serve anyone?

Some Students Do Not Test Well

Every year I ask my college students how many of them are comfortable taking tests. A few hands go up, not many. And when I ask how many feel uncomfortable taking tests, many more hands go up. And sometimes, especially when

I know the group well and they know each other well I will ask, if folks are willing, about test anxiety, and there are always hands that go up. These are college students who succeeded enough in K–12 to not only get into college but also to be headed for a career in teaching, and yet testing is a major issue for many of them. Test anxiety and discomfort are not about intelligence, however that is defined. Many of those who feel uncomfortable with testing or seriously anxious about testing are more than able to demonstrate what they know and understand in other ways.

Multiple intelligence theory also helps us to understand that many of our students are "intelligent" in ways that are missed or ignored through standardized testing, and so when the school system values students only through this one, standardized instrument it is also de-valuing many of our students who can't communicate what they know through a bubble sheet.

The Silence at the Heart of the Education System

Teachers know the harm that is being done by the testing and overwhelmingly oppose it. They know it is poor assessment, that it is biased, that it traumatizes the students and the teachers, that it puts schools in an impossible position, that it interferes with teaching and learning, and yet they feel unable to speak out about it because of fear. They have been ordered to say nothing, to not speak about it; if they do, they may well be disciplined.

Fear now dominates the system. This plays out in several ways, beginning with who gets hired. If a candidate for a building principalship or a district superintendent position is not willing to commit to raising scores as his or her first priority, they are likely not going to be hired for those positions. If they are currently in positions and not sufficiently dedicated to the high-stakes agenda, they are not likely to keep their positions and likely to be frustrated in their attempts to bring more creativity and student-centered approaches to their students. It is a tight fit, a tight spot that administrators find themselves in as the state and the feds apply pressure down the hierarchical ladder.

Principals, in turn hire teachers for their buildings, and they are under that same enormous pressure to hire teachers most likely to raise test scores rather than teachers who will best serve the academic, emotional, and social needs of all their students. And they are under pressure to make sure that teachers are teaching toward the testing throughout the school year, which leads to the kinds of workbook-heavy lessons that we see in too many classrooms, starting in many kindergarten classrooms.

Loss of Local Control

An additional concern related to high-stakes testing is the loss of local control that comes with it. As schools are faced with meeting the testing requirements handed down by federal and state departments of education, they have less room and ability to make decisions at the local level about what to teach and how to teach it. Teachers in many buildings have lost the ability to make decisions about the curriculum they use and the ways they go about meeting the learning needs of their students. Instead they are handed the curriculum they are required to use and the pacing schedule that tells them how fast to move through the curriculum whether the children have mastered the material or not. Administrations at the district and school levels have felt similar pressure to follow the mandates that have been handed down to them and have been constrained from making decisions at the local level. Those who know the children and the communities around the school are able to make fewer and fewer decisions about how to best serve those children and communities, giving over that decision making to bureaucrats who do not know or care about their children or their communities.

A lack of money is another way in which local decision making has been taken from districts and schools. As more and more of what is required of schools is unfunded or underfunded, it leaves the schools without the resources it once had to carry out the educational programs it would like to offer. There is not enough money for science equipment, or field trips, or art supplies, or translators for second-language learners, or adequate supports for students with special needs; that money has gone into meeting the unfunded mandates connected to the testing. Many states are badly underfunding schools, which means that the schools are having to do more with even less. Massachusetts, for example, is currently underfunding its schools by more than a billion dollars (some say by closer to a billion and a half dollars) (Larkin, 2018). This underfunding makes it very difficult for schools to adequately serve their students; costs continually rise and money from the states and the federal government stays relatively flat so that they are forced to continually tighten their belts. With the money they must devote to testing related behaviors, it leaves little money for anything else.

Narrowing Curriculum

When schools devote so much time and money to a testing agenda they are making choices not to spend that time or money on other things. There is almost no social studies in elementary schools. There is less science and almost no hands-on science because it takes too much time and doesn't lead to a "right' answer. There is less art, less music, less recess, fewer group projects, less time for students to explore their interests and questions. All that time has been funneled into a test prep curriculum. There are fewer field trips because field trips take time and involve some expense, and there is no money for that because it is going into testing related purchases or expenses.

Is the focus on test preparation and high-stakes testing worth this trade-off? Are students better prepared to meet a world they can't predict, the world they will be moving into as they move through school and beyond, even if they score well on tests (and they are not scoring any better, as I mentioned above). For those students who are passionate about the arts, about movement, about learning about the world, following their questions and concerns through extended research, what happens to them as they are funneled through a one-size-fits-all chute? Are they better for the experience?

Privateers

Those who want to privatize education are hoping to convince the public that public education is failing and are banking on failing test scores to achieve their aims. The public schools are not failing. The National Assessment of Education Progress (NAEP) scores show that U.S. children are scoring better than they did ten years ago (Hansen et al, 2018), and when we compare U.S. scores with the scores of those in other countries, correcting for the disparities based on poverty, the United States is on par with the best.

The state of New York set out to test all students and announced their "predictions" that only thirty two percent would pass; amazingly enough that's how many passed. The fact that they decided on the cut scores (the score required for passing) after the tests were taken made it easy for them to engineer the results they had predicted. Why would they do this? There is plenty of speculation that the real target is not better education for our children but the 600 billion dollars of public money that goes into public education each year. Private companies would love to get at that money, and one way to do it is to convince the public that their public schools don't work, which could open the door to business moving in to save the day. It is corporate capitalism, barking at the door of democratic education.

Publishing Companies

Publishing companies make hundreds of millions of dollars constructing the tests, publishing the tests, creating textual materials that align with the tests, offering workshops on how to pass the tests, how to teach to the tests, how to remediate students who fail the tests, scoring the tests, creating computer programs that guide students to better scores on tests, creating computer programs to give the tests, and now, creating student-specific programs that address each student's particular learning need. There is a fortune to be made through testing and these private corporations that are only in this for the money are in hot pursuit of those dollars. They are not educators and do not care about the learning the students are or are not learning; in fact, they make more money if the students don't do well and require materials for additional study.

When a state contracts with Pearson, for example, that means that every school in the state is obligated and mandated to buy these Pearson products; they are a "captive market." Consumers (the schools) have no choice but to comply and thus have little to no protection from abuse. They are at the mercy of the supplier. Pearson owns proprietary rights to the testing and scoring, which means no one in the schools gets to see the tests or to question the tests; if they do so they are liable to be sued or disciplined, which is why I was brought up on charges, as I mentioned earlier. No one sees the tests once they are scored, so it is not easy to challenge the scores though there are numerous examples of mistakes made in the scoring process. At the heart of public education is a private, for-profit, noneducational corporation that operates in secret. It is a dream setup for a private corporation; it is a nightmare for a democracy. So why does this happen? Why are things set up this way? Steven Singer says that high stakes testing is

> [...] one of the largest captive markets in existence. That's some 50.4 million children forced to take standardized assessments, created by and marketed by publishing corporations. The largest such corporation, Pearson, boasts profits of $9 billion annually. Its largest competitor, CBT/McGraw-Hill, makes $2 billion annually. Others include Education Testing Services and Riverside Publishing better known through its parent company Houghton Mifflin Harcourt. (Singer, 2017)

Resistance to the Testing: Opting Out

This assault on public education has been met with resistance across the country. It has not been easy, partly because the federal and state governments have been determined not to listen, and partly because educators have been threatened with punishment if they openly oppose the testing policies. This has left it up to independent organizations and parents and families to act against the high-stakes testing policies, and they have done so across the county.

One of the most prominent strategies of resistance against the high-stakes testing policy has been to encourage families to refuse to allow their students to take the test. The legal obligation of the schools is to offer the tests to all their students, but they do not have control over whether the students take the tests; that decision falls within the domain of the parents and guardians of the children.

When I was working at a college in New York State, I worked with a few of my colleagues, parents, and teachers in the community to encourage families in the community to refuse to have their children take the tests as an act of protection for their children and as an act of resistance against federal and state policies that were harmful to public education in the state.

When we began our organizing efforts, there was little interest and little awareness of what was happening in the schools. Families were not hearing any complaints or concerns from their children's teachers and so assumed that nothing had really changed from the time that they had been in school, before No Child Left Behind. They did not realize that the teachers had been ordered to say nothing. That meant that it was left to the public to spread the word.

We organized a public forum at the university so that no district could be identified as trouble makers by the state, which was not happy about these forums designed to help educate the public about their policies. And to be honest, the university was not very happy about our hosting the forum either, afraid that they too would be in trouble with the state. Our group (North Country Allies for Public Education) decided that it was part of the mandate of the university to offer a safe place for the community to come together to discuss important ideas and to help educate each other so we went ahead with the forum.

We talked with a reporter from the local paper, who wrote an advance story about the forum, which helped to educate the public about the issue. We also contacted radio stations in the area and spread the word through flyers, posters, and personal contacts, invited a panel consisting of a local administrator, a local teacher, a local student, a local parent, and a local education professor, all prepared to share their perspective about what was happening in the schools. And then we waited, not knowing if we would be alone in the room or not. It turns out we were not alone.

More than 300 people from communities and school districts across the North Country came to the forum, filling the university lecture hall, and it was amazing. The panel shared their experiences; most riveting was a middle school student who talked about the nonstop testing she was experiencing and the stress that came with it. Once the panel had shared, we opened the floor to anyone who wanted to ask questions or to share their experiences and for the next hour and a half we heard from teachers, administrators, students, and family members expressing their concerns about what was happening in the schools. In all of their schools. That's one of the most powerful aspects of our bringing them together; they had been experiencing their frustration and pain alone, unaware that schools in the next district had the same concerns, frustration, and pain. The power of people coming together was evident, and people left the forum aware that they were not alone, that there were allies, and that they could talk out loud about what was happening.

To make an ongoing and long story short, we went on to hold several more forums over the next two years and our relatively conservative rural North Country community opted out more than sixty percent of their students, making most of the test results statistically invalid (since too few students took the tests), and that percentage has held steady for several years in a row. New York State has had more than 225,000 opt outs a year over the past several years despite threats of consequences from the state, and there have not been any consequences to date.

The high-stakes testing battle is far from over. While No Child Left Behind is no longer the law, having been replaced by ESSA, states are still giving high-stakes tests and insisting that students take them, but resistance continues to grow. Resistance, as they say, is fertile.

There are many organizations working to support resistance to the testing. A few to start with include:

> Fair Test, (fairtest.org) a Boston based national organization that has been working against high stakes testing for many years presents a rationale for why families might want to opt out their children, collects information about resistance efforts going on across the country, presents fact sheets, sample letters, and research supporting resistance to the tests, and serves as a clearing house for groups working across the country.
>
> New York State Allies for Public Education (www.nysape.org), a group that has coordinated and supported opt out and resistance efforts across the state. Their information is useful to anyone, anywhere and includes sample opt out letters, information about how to opt out a student, how to deal with administration, and how to organize with others.

Long Island Opt Out (https://www.facebook.com/groups/Longislandoptout/), a group based in Long Island, NY, that have been leaders in the opt out movement.

United Opt Out (http://www.unitedoptoutnational.org/), a national organization that helps to coordinate and share information from across the country.

References

Au, W. (2009). Unequal by design: High stakes testing and the standardization of inequality. New York: Routledge.

Berliner, D. C. (2009). Poverty and potential: Out-of-school factors and school success. National Education Policy Center. Retrieved from http://nepc.colorado.edu/publication/poverty-and-potential

Hansen, M., Levesque, E. M., Valant, J., & Quintero, D. (2018, June 27). 2018 Brown Center report on American education: Trends in NAEP math, reading, and civics scores. Brookings Institute. Retrieved from https://www.brookings.edu/research/2018-brown-center-report-on-american-education-trends-in-naep-math-reading-and-civics-scores/

Howard, R. & Selwyn, D. (2008). Take this test and …: Doing unto policy makers what they do to students. In Left behind in the race to the top. Gorlewski, J. A. & Pofilio, B. J. editors. pp. 275–286. New York: Pearson.

Larkin, M. (2018, July 11). What's behind the Beacon Hill battle over school funding? WBUR. Retrieved from http://www.wbur.org/edify/2018/07/11/school-funding-bills

Mathewson, T. G. (2017, April 19). How poverty changes the brain. The Atlantic. Retrieved from https://www.theatlantic.com/education/archive/2017/04/can-brain-science-pull-families-out-of-poverty/523479/

Rosner, J. (2003, April 14). On white preference. Nation Magazine, p. 24. Retrieved from http://jayrosner.com/publication-onwhitepreferences.html.

Singer, S. M. (2017, April 8). Standardized testing creates captive markets. Retrieved from https://gadflyonthewallblog.wordpress.com/2017/04/08/standardized-testing-creates-captive-markets/

West, M., quoted in Bergland. (2015, April 18). Why do rich kids have higher standardized test scores? Psychology Today. Retrieved from https://www.psychologytoday.com/us/blog/the-athletes-way/201504/why-do-rich-kids-have-higher-standardized-test-scores

· 8 ·

DENYING OUR CHILDREN

I had the good fortune to teach at all levels of K–12 and so I got to witness the complexities of educating children from kindergarten through high school. We in elementary used to gaze in horror as those children who displayed such joy in our classrooms turned into cynical, jaded middle schoolers and wondered what happened; what were those middle school teachers doing? We in middle school wondered what the elementary teachers were doing such that the students came to us so lacking in so many things, and we gazed in horror at how our lively, loving (though wacky) middle school students became whatever it was they became in high school. And those of us in high school would shake our heads and wonder what had happened at the elementary and middle school levels such that the students who arrived at our doorstep in ninth grade knew so little and were so unready to learn.

After I left K–12 to teach at university I continued to visit the public schools while supervising student teachers and have been on hand to watch the schools change under the weight of No Child Left Behind. It is no longer acceptable to focus on the interests and questions of the children or to spend extended time exploring a topic without a clearly defined "right answer." There is less and less room for children to learn and to demonstrate their learning in ways that match their strengths. And there is much less fun, less joy in learning in the rooms; there isn't time because the tests are waiting.

The increasingly standardized, one-size-fits-all approach to education most in evidence these days actually fits few, as Susan Ohanian named it in her 1999 book. The reality is that while there are students who can do what is asked of them and can pass the tests, they are not well served by a system that does not really care about them as individuals, but only as data points. More and more of our students are being labeled failures, particularly students of color, students living in poverty, students who learn differently than the one-size-fits-all approach employs, and students whose gifts do not match what the school values. We have seen that stress levels are rising in the school house and that schools are not healthy places for an increasing number of children and adults.

I want to briefly address some of the ways in which we have created a system that is failing our children by denying them essential aspects of who they are. We are robbing them of a sense of belonging, a sense of meaning, and the confidence and skills they need to live happy, healthy, successful lives.

Denying Their Language

Many Native Americans were literally forbidden to speak their languages at school after they had been removed from reservations and taken to boarding schools in order to "kill the Indian to save the man," to quote Richard Pratt, the founder of the Carlisle Indian School. Tommy Porter, an Iroquois elder, tells the story of his experience at boarding school, where there was a conscious effort to eradicate the Mohawk language, religion, and culture. These were government schools, but the teachers were all Christians.

> "Don't talk Mohawk." [...] I was attacked all the time. My language was attacked in school, year after year, and I was punished for it. There was no place there for the things in the Longhouse that I have. When we tried it we were reprimanded for it. [...] Our music, our art, our baskets, or anything we did that was artistic was forbidden in there. Even our story, our history. (Porter, 2008, 28)

This experience at school put Tommy Porter and his classmates in an impossible situation. Their families and community and their elders were educating them about the world as they knew and experienced it, and their school was telling them that what they were hearing from their own families and communities was wrong. There was no win in this situation; only loss.

> But I'm not immune to colonization either, 'cause I was just a kid. So, one of the things that hurts me so bad I still can't even deal with it is … I had good teachers, *good teachers*: Grandma and Grandpa and all of them […] And they told me things, and then the school told me not to believe them because they weren't "documented." What I'm saying to you is that no white man, nobody foreign is there anymore twisting my arm or kicking my butt as they did when I was a kid. Not *anymore*.
>
> Because now the image of that person is in here, in my head, way subconsciously kicking my butt every day. *I'm kicking my own butt*. So, no physical American or Canadian man has to do it to me anymore. He's already inside here where I can't get him out. That's what they call the colonization process. That's how effective it is. It's deadly. (Porter, 2008, 30–31)

While what happened to Tommy Porter and his classmates happened some time ago, the practice of denying language is still happening in our schools. Lisa Delpit talks of the role that identity plays with relation to language and that when students are always corrected for speaking in what is sometimes called Ebonics, the language and dialect they speak at home and in their community, it is an assault on their culture and identity. In response to a question about what teachers should do in relation to the so-called Ebonics debate she says,

> First, they should recognize that the linguistic form a student brings to school is intimately connected with loved ones, community, and personal identity. To suggest that this form is wrong, or, even worse, ignorant is to suggest that something is wrong with the student and his or her family. (Delpit, 2009)

There are also numerous incidents in which students speaking Spanish in class to each other are disciplined, ordered to "speak American." A video clip of a teacher saying this to students in a New Jersey high school went viral in 2017 (Benavides, 2017), but this incident was not the only case of students being disciplined and/or forbidden to speak their home language in class (Mathews, 2013).

The settings in which students attend school can cause them to be caught in the middle of two worlds, with an either implied or stated judgment that their home, culture, and community are somehow inferior, which pushes some students to rebellion, some to compliance, some to withdrawal and that pushes all away from wholeness, from health. An essential part of them has been labeled not good enough, and the strong bonds of love and trust between them and their families are undermined by authorities who hold their educational futures in their control.

Denying Their Language and Culture

Precious Knowledge (Palos, 2011) is a film that documents a Mexican American studies program in Tucson, Arizona, focused on offering students a place to learn about their history and culture. Tucson was a part of Mexico before the United States stole what is now the entire U.S. Southwest in the 1840s via a manufactured war with Mexico. Those who had been Mexican citizens suddenly became foreigners, illegal immigrants in a foreign country without moving a muscle or taking a step. For the students in Tucson, the course in Mexican American history was a chance to become healthier, more whole, to value and learn about who they were and the history and culture that brought them to this point. What they learned in other classes was centered on the European American experience, through a European American lens. Having students learn about their culture and history in this program served them well; their graduation rates and attendance were higher than their peers who were not in the program.

The students in the Mexican American studies classroom, taught by Curtis Acosta and Jose Gonzalez, learned about their own culture, history, and language, and then worked together to understand how that past informs their present. The program was shut down by the state superintendent of education and other politicians who said it was teaching the students to hate whites and was anti-American, but that ruling was challenged in court by Acosta and students in the program and, after several years of court proceedings, the students won their suit. The court ruled that the Mexican American studies program had been shut down because of "racial animus," and there was no justification for doing so.

We attended an event that featured young students of color talking about their experiences in middle and high school and it was disturbing. The students said they felt dismissed, discounted, and discouraged by teachers who had no time for them, by classmates who rejected them for their skin color or language, and by a disciplinary system that disproportionately found them to be the problem, even when they were clearly defending themselves from abuse brought to them by their white peers.

Each of the young people speaking at the session somehow felt a failure, that it was something they did that was not good enough or that caused the problem, and while the adults in the room were quick to reassure them that there was nothing wrong with them, that does not solve the problem. How do we expect our children to learn and to be healthy when they are denied who they are and surrounded by hate and rejection and treated as less than equal by those in charge of their education and well-being?

What we are seeing at the southern border, with young children being separated from their families and put in cages by an administration that came to power largely based on racist rhetoric, is a tragedy and horror that highlights the strong current of racism that continues to run through the country and that continues to bring harm and violence to students of color in our schools when that is part of their daily experience.

Home Values and Expectations Conflict With School Values and Expectations

Denying students their culture is not only about their history. When there is a large gap between what is valued at home and the community and what is valued by the school, students can be caught here too. Maria Timmons Flores talks about this gap experienced by migrant workers from Mexico, working in the Pacific Northwest:

> Family comes first. If your family needs to support itself, you do whatever you need to do to support your family. Kids work in the fields when they are twelve, watch their younger brothers and sisters. We see seven-year olds watching two and three-year olds … you bring them to the fields with you where they hang out all day. It's for survival.
>
> So, part of it is about family, and what do I need to do to help my family survive. But part of it is, if you talk to the kids, schools are not healthy or happy places for them. They are talented and capable but given the demands placed on them in a school context that is not supportive, they are unable to achieve their potential—it's the opportunity gap. If you get the message every day that there is something wrong with you, and your family, or something wrong with the way you speak, or you try as hard as you can and you can't possibly be successful, you're a lot happier being in the fields with your family, where you are working, playing in the fields with your friends, having a meal with your family, and that's what you know, that's where you come from. To me, it's a really rational, human choice. Where can I go to make a contribution, to be with people who love and support me, a place where I feel good. If we are thinking about how we create healthy children, unless as a society we disrupt the conditions we put children and families in, we can't possibly change things. (Maria Timmons Flores, Personal communication, 2016)

I had a chance to communicate again with Dr. Flores in 2018 and she added this comment.

> Although immigration has always been a traumatizing threat for mixed immigration status families—the fear that you will return from school to find a parent

> deported—in these times this is a palpable fear that children experience every day. Under the current administration, family separation is an ever-present fear everywhere, not just on the border. Even young children experience the hatred behind anti-immigrant rhetoric, policies, practices. (Flores, 2018, Personal communication)

The same could be said for the experiences of students from various Asian populations. They and their ancestors have been labeled/portrayed/stereotyped in ways that are historically inaccurate, demeaning, and exclusionary, giving students the clear message that they don't really belong, and that in fact they are threats to the well-being of the country. This has been an ongoing theme through U.S. history. The United States excluded Chinese in the 1880s, limited the number of Japanese immigrants in the so-called gentleman's agreement in the early 1900s, and in the 1920s Japanese, Korean, and Chinese were denied citizenship or naturalization, were prevented from marrying Caucasians, and were not allowed to own land. There were violent attacks on Filipinos in the 1930s, and the United States incarcerated more than 120,000 Japanese Americans as potential threats during World War II despite there being no evidence to suggest they were working with "the enemy." Many people from the countries of Southeast Asia faced hatred and discrimination when they came here to escape possible imprisonment and death following what is known in the United States as the Vietnam War in the 1960s and 1970s.

And little needs to be said about the ways in which Muslim Americans have been treated in the first two decades of the twenty-first century, from the burning of or desecration of mosques to the attacks on women wearing the hijab, to physical violence aimed at Muslims; the United States has not been a safe or welcoming or healthy place for Muslims to be.

Denying Point of View

Howard Zinn titled his personal memoir *You Can't Be Neutral on a Moving Train* and makes the point throughout that there is no such thing as neutrality when we look at history. We all come from our histories, our experiences, our neighborhoods, and they all shape who we are and how we see the world. When schools insist that what they are getting from their state-supplied curriculum guides and from their textbooks is neutral and that anything else is biased, they are engaging in a lie that often contradicts the views and values of the students in the room. The official story is not neutral or unbiased;

decisions are made about what to include, what to omit, whose voices to feature, and whose stories to tell, and those decisions are made based on many points of view: the members of the curriculum committee at the table, the textbook manufacturers, those sensitive to the political winds, and so on. It is not possible to be neutral in these cases, and one of the fundamental lies that has been told about U.S. history is that there is a neutral, "just the facts ma'am" version of what has happened in the world. Paulo Freire spoke of how this approach serves the state:

> Just as there are no neutral city or state administrations, there are no neutral educational systems. It is impossible for me to think about education without considering the question of power, of asking the question: In favor of whom or what do we promote education? In the United States it is necessary to negate the political nature of education to give the superficial appearance that education serves everyone. But the more you deny the political dimension of education, the more you assume the potential to blame the victims—the dropouts are to blame. And the dropouts, for the most part, are from "minority" groups ... When curriculum designers fail to incorporate "minority" groups' values in the curriculum, when they refuse to accept and legitimize the students' language, their actions point to the inflexibility, insensitivity and rigidity of a curriculum designed to benefit those who wrote it. (Freire and Macedo, 1987)

It is not only state education committees that are deciding on the curriculum our children will be experiencing. Harriot (2018) reports that this ideological assault through control of the curriculum is still very much with us. The Koch brothers are funding the distribution of social studies materials, for free, that glorifies the free market, that whitewashes African American history, and that praises the ideas of small government in service to the most important members of society, the property owners. The lessons stress limited government, religious freedom [for Christians, author], free-market economics and—worst of all—a revisionist version of the history of slavery that paints it as a necessary evil to further freedom and democracy

The lessons are appalling, cherry-picking historical documents in such a slanted way that millions of young people are going to come out of their schooling knowing less about their history than they went in, and what they "know" will be right wing doctrine as interpreted by the Koch brothers. And who will buy this crap? Districts that have been starved to the point of desperation, districts that can't afford textbooks or curriculum committees or much of anything else, or districts run by ideologically conservative school boards. These same districts may no longer have a curriculum coordinator, a luxury they can no longer afford, so there is less quality control and coordination concerning what is taught.

And then there's Texas.

> This fall, Texas schools will teach students that Moses played a bigger role in inspiring the Constitution than slavery did in starting the Civil War, ignoring the *Declaration of the Immediate Causes Which Induce and Justify the Secession of South Carolina from the Federal Union* (1860), which states clearly that they seceded over the issue of slavery. The Lone Star State's new social studies textbooks, deliberately written to play down slavery's role in Southern history, do not threaten only Texans—they pose a danger to schoolchildren all over the country.
>
> The Texas board of education adopted a revised social studies curriculum in 2010 after a fierce battle. When it came to social studies standards, conservatives championing causes from a focus on the biblical underpinnings of our legal system to a whitewashed picture of race in the United States won out. The guidelines for teaching Civil War history were particularly concerning: They teach that "sectionalism, states' rights and slavery"—carefully ordered to stress the first two and shrug off the last—caused the conflict. (Washington Post Editorial Board, 2015)

In this time where more and more of our actual information is labeled fake news, where the president is willing to say anything to anyone, even if it contradicts what he said to someone else an hour ago, our students are in grave danger of having no idea of where they have come from or why things are the way they are.

The consequence of denying students who they are is alienation and withdrawal. They stop asking questions because they know they will not get real answers, or the answers they get will be at odds with what they are hearing from their families, from their communities, and from other texts or sources.

Denying the Reality of Maturation and Development

We each grow and develop at our own rates. While there are general guidelines and benchmarks about who five-year-olds are, these are just that, general guidelines rather than indications of ideal rates of growth and maturation. My parents tell me that I was a late walker and began my locomotion by crawling backward, perhaps a clue as to what was to come. There are many benchmarks that new parents look for in their newborns, and some become anxious when their child does not lift her head on the day that books or internet articles suggest is *the* day for that to happen. Hopefully, after speaking with doctors, with other new parents, and maybe with their own parents, they come to realize that there is a uniqueness to the pace of development.

We do want to have a general set of guidelines to help us identify what may be a problem; if there is a wide variance between our child and what is a normal benchmark for turning over or walking, we may want to investigate why this is so. The same is true as children get older; there is not one "right" answer to where a five-year-old or a fifteen-year-old should be developmentally, but there is a general range outside of which we may want to begin paying closer attention to make sure there are no underlying issues that need attention.

Development is a complex process, and while we tend to focus on particular benchmarks or passages, there are actually several areas developing at the same time, some more visible and apparent than others. The University of Washington child development department identifies five different areas developing all at once in young children: physical, intellectual, social, emotional, and moral, and we are all a mix of those areas (University of Washington, n.d.). Some develop more quickly physically, others more socially, some intellectually; they don't all happen at the same pace. We are all influenced by our genetics and our environment, both nature and nurture. We want to pay attention to what we are noticing, being aware of differences without judging or coming to quick conclusions, while recognizing that some children may need more support in certain areas than do others.

Ken Robinson (Robinson and Aronica, 2015) labels the approach to education that treats all students as if they have the same experience, develop at the same rate, and are responsible for the same product or output as an industrial approach. We treat education as we might an assembly line; all students go through the same sequence in the same way, as we turn them into completed products at graduation. This standardized approach is more harmful to some than it is to others, but it is not good for anyone.

There is a real danger that some students will get lost, and there will be students who are not getting what they need; they may be students who have completed assignments by the time the teacher is done passing them out, or students who need more time, or students who really want to process the material more deeply, or students who are passionate about some topic that is not aligned with the one-size-fits-all curriculum. It may seem easier and less messy if everyone does the same thing at the same time, but it does not serve the real learning needs of students, and it makes it more difficult to reach the full range of learners.

For me, moving into more of a student-centered approach that gave room for group work and a variety of responses to assignments helped me to get to know the students more personally, and what they did with their projects made them more real to me as individuals. It made my teaching more effective and enjoyable for the students and more successful for me than it would have been taking a more traditional march through the textbook chapters and questions, with everyone doing the same thing at the same time in the same way. It was also a bonus to not have to read 150 of the exact same essays at a time.

When we ignore who children are and what they care about, and when we don't respect the ways in which they learn we are teaching them to deny themselves, to learn to not listen to themselves, which comes with a cost. A psychological cost, a social cost, an emotional cost as well as an academic cost. When we standardize our classrooms and expect that all students behave in the same way it is a problem. We hope our children grow and develop into people who are independent thinkers and actors who can make good decisions based on a clear sense of what is right and yet we give them little opportunity to develop those decision-making skills in classrooms that are regimented and industrialized. There is very little thinking that goes on along the assembly line, by design. Your job isn't to think, it is to weld the bumper onto the car, over and over again. So it is with standardized education.

Denying Play

As mentioned earlier, when young children are forced to spend long hours sitting in front of workbooks, part of what they are losing is the time to play. Play is a crucial aspect of how young students learn about themselves and about the world.

> Young children work hard at play. They invent scenes and stories, solve problems, and negotiate their way through social roadblocks. They know what they want to do and work diligently to do it. Because their motivation comes from within, they learn the powerful lesson of pursuing their own ideas to a successful conclusion.
>
> Research shows that children who engage in complex forms of socio-dramatic play have greater language skills than nonplayers, better social skills, more empathy, more imagination, and more of the subtle capacity to know what others mean. They are less aggressive and show more self-control and higher levels of thinking. Animal research suggests that they have larger brains with more complex neurological structures than nonplayers. Long-term research casts doubt on the assumption that starting earlier on the teaching of phonics and other discrete skills leads to better results. (Miller and Almon, 2009, 7)

> China and Japan are envied in the U.S. for their success in teaching science, math, and technology. But one rarely hears about their approach to schooling before second grade, which is playful and experiential rather than didactic. Finland's children, too, go to playful kindergartens, and they enter first grade at age seven rather than six. They enjoy a lengthy, playful early childhood. (Miller and Almon, 2009, 8)

The teacher has a crucial role in a child-centered classroom, attending to the serious work the children are exploring through their play and supporting it by providing appropriate materials, by providing the time and space for the children to engage in play, and by resisting the pressure to fast track five-year-olds into college preparatory programs. When children are forced to sit for long periods of time with workbooks rather than engaging in movement and play, they are violating what they are developmentally ready to do and are forcing their bodies to do what they are not ready for, at the expense of their health and development. B. F. Skinner showed that you can train pigeons to do what pigeons are not trained to do, but does that help them to be better pigeons?

Laura Weldon says that children who are forced to read too early, before they are ready, are actually working against what their bodies are able to do:

> In order for children to read, write and spell they must be developmentally ready. Some are ready at the age of four or five, some not for *many* years later. This readiness includes complex neurological pathways and kinesthetic awareness. It includes the proprioceptive sense developed through sensory receptors in the muscles, joints, and tendons: a form of maturation essential for a physical sense of self (even essential for learning how to modulate one's voice and to hold objects carefully).
>
> Such readiness isn't created by workbooks or computer programs. It's the result of brain maturation as well as rich experiences found in bodily sensation and movement. (Weldon, 2012)

Occupational therapist Angela Hanscom says that children are not spending enough time playing, not moving enough. Hanscom says,

> We need to fix the underlying issue. Recess times need to be extended and kids should be playing outside as soon as they get home from school. Twenty minutes of movement a day is not enough! They need hours of play outdoors in order to establish a healthy sensory system and to support higher-level attention and learning in the classroom.
>
> In order for children to learn, they need to be able to pay attention. In order to pay attention, we need to let them move. (Hanscom, 2014)

Denying the Ways That People Learn

I have asked audiences in many different settings and contexts whether those with siblings or those with more than one child would say that the children were alike enough that there would be one teaching approach or one assessment that would adequately capture/reflect who they are, and no one has ever said yes. They laugh and start to tell stories about how different they are from their siblings, or how they have one child who does this while the other child (or children) in the family is (are) so very different—which makes sense; we clearly share genetic material and similar nurture from our families, but we are unique individuals. My three stepchildren are all very bright, passionate, caring people who carry many of the characteristics of their parents, and yet in many ways they are not alike at all. They are not well served by the same approaches, learning systems, or structures, which might explain why our house meetings were the way they were.

This is only a problem or concern if your goal is to have children fit identically into a "learning" box much like cans of soup or sardines, where having containers all the same size and shape makes for easy packaging and stacking. When we try to do that with our children in school settings, making life easier for us as educators, we find out very quickly that some don't fit in that box. As Ken Robinson put it, what children in first grade have in common is their date of manufacture, and not necessarily much else. What does this mean for us in education, and what impact does this insistence on an industrial approach to schooling have on the health and well-being of our children?

Multiple Intelligences

This also becomes an issue when we think about how people learn and process information. Howard Gardner challenged the belief that it is possible to measure intelligence and assign a definitive number to it. Gardner, a psychologist, developed the theory of multiple intelligences after working with patients who had suffered brain injuries. He found that injuries to certain parts of the brain corresponded to loss of certain functions, but that those patients retained abilities in other areas. Gardner originally identified seven (then eight, and now nine) discreet areas of intelligence that he said we all had, to one degree or another. The intelligences briefly described are:

- VISUAL/SPATIAL—children who learn best visually and organizing things spatially. They like to see what you are talking about in order to understand. They enjoy charts, graphs, maps, tables, illustrations, art, puzzles, costumes—anything eye-catching.
- VERBAL/LINGUISTIC—children who demonstrate strength in the language arts: speaking, writing, reading, listening. These students have always been successful in traditional classrooms because their intelligence lends itself to traditional teaching.
- MATHEMATICAL/LOGICAL—children who display an aptitude for numbers, reasoning, and problem solving. This is the other half of the children who typically do well in traditional classrooms where teaching is logically sequenced, and students are asked to conform.
- BODILY/KINESTHETIC—children who experience learning best through activity: games, movement, hands-on tasks, building. These children were often labeled "overly active" in traditional classrooms where they were told to sit and be still!
- MUSICAL/RHYTHMIC—children who learn well through songs, patterns, rhythms, instruments, and musical expression. It is easy to overlook children with this intelligence in traditional education.
- INTRAPERSONAL—children who are especially in touch with their own feelings, values, and ideas. They may tend to be more reserved, but they are actually quite intuitive about what they learn and how it relates to themselves.
- INTERPERSONAL—children who are noticeably people oriented and outgoing and do their learning cooperatively in groups or with a partner. These children may have typically been identified as "talkative" or "too concerned about being social" in a traditional setting.
- NATURALIST—children who love the outdoors, animals, field trips. More than this, though, these students love to pick up on subtle differences in meanings. The traditional classroom has not been accommodating to these children.
- EXISTENTIALIST—children who learn in the context of where humankind stands in the "big picture" of existence. They ask, "Why are we here?" and "What is our role in the world?" This intelligence is seen in the discipline of philosophy.

A person who is very "intelligent" in math may be less "intelligent" in one of the other eight areas of intelligence. While we have always known that each of us has strengths and weaknesses (please don't let me work on repairing my car or, more importantly, yours), what is different about Gardner's work is that it raises all nine areas to the same plane of importance and value, challenging and supplanting the view that there is a single, measurable intelligence that is most highly valued and other, lesser skills that people have. Schools tend to favor or privilege certain of these nine intelligences so that some students strong in those areas do well while others, who are stronger in other intelligences tend to struggle, but this does not mean those who struggle are less intelligent; their strengths do not align with what the school system has chosen to value.

IQ and the Eugenics Movement

This idea of a single, measurable intelligence came out of the American eugenics movement of the early 1900s, pushed by Lewis Terman, of Stanford University, among others. Terman took the Binet test that had been developed in France to help address the needs of specific children with learning challenges and transformed it into the Stanford Binet Intelligence test, a "scientific" instrument that he claimed could accurately measure intelligence in the general population. Terman and others in the eugenics movement believed that there was a superior race surrounded by inferior races, and he wanted to use the Stanford Binet test to help sort the wheat from the chaff, so to speak, and to spend time and resources educating those most able to learn (white, western, and northern Europeans) rather than wasting time on those who could not learn beyond a very basic level (African-Americans, Latinx, Native Americans, southern Europeans). Schools tended to be designed to serve those of the "superior" race, catering to the approaches and expectations most in line with their cultural ways of being. This placed those who learned and moved through the world differently at a disadvantage.

Eugenicists further believed that the lesser races passed on inferior or "defective" genes that resulted in criminality, poverty, and other crimes. They wanted to limit the spread of these defective genes and succeeded in convincing more than thirty state legislatures into passing involuntary sterilization laws that targeted "defective strains" within the general population (Bouche and Rivard, 2014). On the national level, eugenics supporters played a decisive role in the congressional passage of the draconian Immigration and Restriction Act of 1924, which established blatantly racist quotas. President Calvin Coolidge embraced the eugenic assumptions behind the law when he declared, "America must be kept American. Biological laws show that Nordics deteriorate when mixed with other races" (Stoskopf, 2012, 35).

The current administration's policies on immigration, from travel bans, to separating families and caging the children, to inflammatory rhetoric, to the Make America Great Again/America First slogans, suggest that the eugenics movement is still alive and has a friend in this administration.

Standardized Education: Working on the Assembly Line

Treating or attempting to treat all our learners as if they were standardized is a losing game, and those who lose most are the children who are most distant from some mythical norm or standard. Those who learn differently, those whose learning strengths are not reading and writing, those who need to move and work with their hands to best learn, those who are learning in a second language, and those who have learning challenges often find that they are "square pegs" who don't fit into the "round holes," and that the system is not designed to serve them any more than a factory is designed to deal with products on the assembly line that don't meet their manufacturing standards. In a factory, those items that don't meet standards are disposed of as waste in the manufacturing process.

If It's 10:30 It Must Be Math

Schools have been organized around what are known as Carnegie Units, created in the late nineteenth and early twentieth centuries that dictated what students were required to complete during their schooling to earn their diploma. The requirements were based on seat time, the amount of time children spent in English class, for example, and led schools to create the daily schedules that continue to this day, more than a century later. Teachers learn to design their lessons to fit into this prefab period of time, rather than to take the time necessary to teach the content of the day's lesson.

As Dennis Littky puts in a TED Talk when describing the multiperiod, disconnected day that most high schoolers live through,

> If you were teaching your own kid at home you wouldn't put him in the living room for forty-five minutes, then ring a bell and bring him into the bathroom so you could do science […] you wouldn't do it that way, it's ridiculous. (https://www.youtube.com/watch?v=UbpqVPtUIFQ)

George Wood, a long-time principal in Ohio, encouraged his staff to shadow students through their typical day to better understand what it was like for them, as part of his plan to bring change to his school:

> Teachers, faced with mountains of material to cover and very little time to cover it, resort to lecture to try and hit the high points. When students tell us they are bored and that the curriculum is incoherent to them, it is to this that they are referring [...] Because we have decided to break curriculum into small, disconnected bits and attempt to cover more information than is reasonably possible, school seems to most students to be a never-ending listing of stuff to jot down, memorize, feedback on a test, and forget. (Wood, 2005, 18)

For young people in middle school and high school (especially) who are social beings, very connected to peers, we allow them little or no time to connect with others, which is what is most important to them. Three or four minutes between classes, which means passing through crowded hallways, saying brief hellos to friends, perhaps a stop at a locker or the rest room, and then beating the bell into a class dedicated to "something completely different," as the Monty Pythons said it, works against who they are and sets many up for alienation if not failure. The more we view children as wild animals that need to be broken and tamed, working against their emotional and intellectual developmental stages, the more we are compromising their potential investment and involvement in making meaning from their experiences.

Students Are Denied Hope, Meaning, and Joy

Finally, students are being denied any hope of making meaning from their time at school or of finding joy and excitement related to learning. When everything is determined by others, from what is studied, to how it is studied, to when it is studied and the pace of that study, and then to how it is assessed, students learn that their own voices, views, and values don't matter. And when they are denied their language, their culture, their history, their interests, and their voices, it becomes clear that the only meaning they can make is that they don't matter. They learn to keep their heads down and conform, they disrupt and challenge, or they drop out. A few weeks ago, a very right wing talk show host took basketball player LeBron James to task for speaking up about his concerns and told him that he was a basketball player and that he should shut up and dribble. That's essentially the message given to our students from this approach to teaching and learning; shut up and bubble.

Emma Gonzalez is one of the students from Parkland, Florida, where the school shooting that took seventeen lives took place. Emma and several of her classmates have been speaking out for gun control and calling out legislators and others who have been unwilling to act for stricter gun control, to act to keep our young people safe.

> "If you have ever lost someone very important to you, then you already know how it feels, and if you haven't, then you cannot possibly imagine it," wrote Lemony Snicket in *The Bad Beginning: A Series of Unfortunate Events*. There are people who do not know, and will never know, what it feels like to go through this. For that I am eternally thankful. But to the people out there who disagree with us: if you have ever felt what it's like to deal with all of this, you would know we aren't doing this for attention. If these funerals were for your friends, you would know this grief is real, not paid for. We are children who are being expected to act like adults, while the adults are proving themselves to behave like children.
>
> When did *children* become such a dirty word? Adults are saying that children are lazy, meanwhile Jaclyn Corin organized an entire trip to Tallahassee, three busses stuffed with 100 kids and reporters who went to discuss our pitiful firearm legislation with the people who can—but won't—do something about it.
>
> Adults are saying that children are emotional. I should hope so—some of our closest friends were taken before their time because of a senseless act of violence that should never have occurred. If we weren't emotional, they would criticize us for that, as well. Adults are saying that children are disrespectful. But how can we respect people who don't respect us? We have always been told that if we see something wrong, we need to speak up; but now that we are, all we're getting is disrespect from the people who made the rules in the first place. Adults like us when we have strong test scores, but they hate us when we have strong opinions. (Gonzalez, 2018)

References

Benavides, C. (2017, October 16). Students walk out after teacher orders: Speak 'American'. NBC news. Retrieved from https://www.nbcnews.com/news/latino/students-walk-out-after-teacher-tells-students-speak-american-n811256

Bouche, T. & Rivard, L. (2014, September 18). America's hidden history: The eugenics movement. Scitable by Nature Education. Retrieved from https://www.nature.com/scitable/forums/genetics-generation/america-s-hidden-history-the-eugenics-movement-123919444.

Delpit, L. (2009). Ebonics and culturally responsive instruction. In Rethinking multicultural education (W. Au, ed). pp. 121–129. Milwaukee: Rethinking Schools.

Flores, M. T. (2016). Personal communication.

Flores, M. T. (2018). Personal communication.

Freire, P. & Macedo, D. (1987). Literacy: Reading the word and the world. South Hadley, MA: Bergin & Garvey.

Gardner, H. (n.d.) Multiple intelligences. Retrieved from http://web.cortland.edu/andersmd/learning/MI%20Theory.htm

Gonzalez, E. (2018, February 26). Parkland student Emma González opens up about her fight for gun control. Harper's Bazaar. Retrieved from https://www.harpersbazaar.com/culture/politics/a18715714/protesting-nra-gun-control-true-story/

Hanscom, A. (2014, July 8). Why so many kids can't sit still in school today. Washington Post. Retrieved from https://www.washingtonpost.com/news/answer-sheet/wp/2014/07/08/why-so-many-kids-cant-sit-still-in-school-today/?utm_term=.f20bc356ee67

Harriot, M. (2018, March 14). Millions of students are quietly being taught the Koch brothers' whitewashed version of Black history. The Root. Retrieved from https://www.theroot.com/millions-of-students-are-quietly-being-taught-the-koch-1823742091

Littky, D. (2011, March 5). Ted talk. You tube. Retrieved from https://www.youtube.com/watch?v=UbpqVPtUIFQ

Mathews, K. (2013, December 7). 5 schools that tried to ban speaking Spanish. Care2. Retrieved from https://www.care2.com/causes/5-schools-that-tried-to-ban-speaking-spanish.html

Miller, E. & Almon, J. (2009). Crisis in the kindergarten: Why children need to play in school. College Park, MD: Alliance for Childhood.

Palos, A. L. (2011). Precious Knowledge. DVD.

Porter, T. (2008). And grandma said …: Iroquois teachings passed down through the oral tradition. Bloomington, Indiana: Xlibris Publishing.

Palso, A. L. (2011). Precious Knowledge DVD.

Robinson, K. & Aronica, L. (2015). Creative schools: The grassroots revolution that's transforming education. New York: Viking.

Stoskopf, A. (2012). Racism in the history of standardized testing: Legacies for today. In Pencils Down (W. Au and M. B. Temple, eds). pp. 34–40. Milwaukee: Rethinking Schools.

University of Washington. (n.d.). Developmental stages.

Washington Post Editorial Board. (2015, July 6). How Texas is whitewashing Civil War history. Washington Post. Retrieved from https://www.washingtonpost.com/opinions/whitewashing-civil-war-history-for-young-minds/2015/07/06/1168226c-2415-11e5-b77f-eb13a215f593_story.html?utm_term=.e5d14218e687

Weldon, L. G. (2012, August 7). Reading readiness has to do with the body. Retrieved from https://lauragraceweldon.com/2012/08/07/reading-readiness-has-to-do-with-the-body/

Wood, G. (2005). Time to learn: How to create high schools that serve all students. Portsmouth, NH: Heinemann

Zinn, H. (2002). You can't be neutral on a moving train: A personal history of our times. Boston, MA: Beacon.

· 9 ·

WHAT CAN SCHOOLS DO?

Schools can and do play a significant role in supporting the health and well-being of our children. The children are in school five days a week, six hours a day, and the influences, opportunities, and connections students make during those hours can have a profound impact on the quality of their lives. We know that children bring their worlds with them when they walk into classrooms, and as we have seen in previous chapters, those worlds contain much that potentially undermines their health. Key aspects of each teacher's work are to assess each child academically, and to also assess them emotionally and socially. She then can organize her work such that all students are getting what they most need in all areas. To remind me of this responsibility and focus I posted a list of guiding questions to consider when I sat down to plan lessons and units. The questions were: Who are the children, and what strengths do they bring? What challenges (academic, social, emotional) do the students bring with them into the classroom? In what ways am I responding to the students and their challenges? What is most important for the students to gain from their time with me this year? In what ways are my actions aligned with what I say I value most? How can we learn with as much joy and engagement as possible? These questions helped me to keep my focus on the whole child, and not to limit my focus to the academic content we were supposed to cover.

Each teacher and school must find ways to stay focused on what matters most to them, on what helps them to best serve their students. I will explore in this chapter some of the things schools either are doing or could do to support and sustain the health of our children as examples of what is possible. The examples are not presented as recipes to be followed, but hopefully as suggestions and/or reminders of steps we can take in schools to improve the health and education of our children.

I've organized a long list of things schools do (or could do) to support the health of children into four general areas: relationships/emotional support, physical health, opportunity to grow/expand, and learning how to learn. There is much overlap among them, but they allow for an exploration of how schools do what they do, and to explore what more they can do to support or children.

Many of the practices and examples I will be sharing in this chapter are relatively simple and straightforward, and many of them may well be already happening in the school buildings around you. I am sharing them as examples of steps that teachers or schools can take that don't depend on a large influx of money or resources; many are steps that can be taken tomorrow. I hope and trust that educators and schools will not stop with these suggestions but will work together to move beyond them to the most effective actions you can take in your school.

Relationships

Everyone I spoke with and everything I read places relationships as the most significant of the factors that make it possible for students to be healthy, happy, and academically successful. There needs to be someone who absolutely believes in and advocates for each student and will stand with them no matter what. Often that person is someone in the family, or community, but for students to be successful in the school setting there must also be someone at school who can be trusted, who listens, and who will stand up for and with each student.

Adults can offer love and security, a sense of belief in the capability and value of the child, and who can serve as a model and mentor, and open doors to the larger, wider world. It is this role, more than any other, that is within our reach as school workers. This is true no matter how many resources the school does or does not have, and it is of fundamental importance to all students, no matter their circumstances. When we treat students with respect, when we help them make connections between their homes, communities, and school, when we help them to make meaning for themselves, we are serving them well. We can develop these relationships in many ways.

Educator Deborah Meier is concerned that adults have in many ways vanished from the lives of our children, leaving them "adrift, without the support or nurturance of grown-ups, without the surrounding of a community in which they might feel safe to try out various roles, listen into the world of adults …" (Meier, 2002, 12). It did not used to be like that, says Meier, as "children once learned the arts and crafts of being a grown-up by belonging to a community whose habits and rituals they naturally absorbed." (2002, 11). They spent more time with adults, in apprenticeships, in multiage settings, working in the family business, so that they saw what it meant to be an adult, for better and worse, and had a sense of what lay ahead for them. Society has changed and there is less certainty for young people in terms of what awaits them; fewer are simply going into the family business, and there are fewer structured times for them to be in the company of adults.

Anthropologist Richard Robbins is also concerned about this, fearing that we have essentially left our children in the care of media, which does not have their interests at heart, and in the care of each other.

> I think we treat our children terribly. Their major babysitter is television. The economic system requires now, usually, two incomes which immediately changes the dynamics of the family. Child care facilities are abysmal, generally, so the whole system is not geared towards producing well-being. Not at all. It's geared toward warehousing the kids and relieving the parents of some of their responsibilities so that they can, by necessity, go earn the money they need to maintain the standards of living that's becoming harder and harder to maintain.
>
> So, what we have essentially done in our society, we have turned our kids over to the marketers, on the one hand, and on the other hand to their peers, who are also, by and large being controlled by the marketers. So, you get all the issues that surround that, class issues, gender issues. Television is particularly saturated with gender issues. (Richard Robbins, 2017, personal communication)

This makes even more important the role that teachers play as adults who forge meaningful relationships with the children they work with, offering support, mentoring, modeling, and a place for conversation.

There are many ways to go about doing this. It is potentially easier in the elementary grades, where a teacher is with her students for most of the day, but even then, with twenty-five or more in a room there are often children who do not experience the trust and closeness that is so central to a child feeling she belongs and is valued. Building trust and relationships take time and attention; they don't happen automatically. They happen in small steps beginning on the first day of school, or sometimes even before the school year starts.

Connections Between the Schools and the Community

Connections between the schools and homes begin when the children begin pre-school, or kindergarten. Hopefully these connections will become the foundation of an alliance and friendship between families and the schools. The contacts can begin through home visits, before school gatherings, in school orientations, or even through phone calls. What matters is that there is the beginning of a relationship between the teacher and family, however that can happen.

Home Visits

One step that some teachers take is to visit students and families before the school year starts. This accomplishes many things: it tells the child and her family that the teacher is willing to take the time to reach out in this way, that she cares enough to make the visit. It helps the teacher to see the context in which her students live, and to get to know a bit more about their culture and setting. The teacher begins to develop a relationship with the family, establishing a baseline understanding that she and the family are in this together for the good of the child. The family can communicate what they think is most important, what their concerns may be, and to help their teacher know more about their child. It's always best when first contacts with families are positive, and not because the child is in trouble. They have that beginning relationship and understanding to build on if there comes a time when the child has an issue at school that needs to be discussed, and hopefully the parents/family members will have enough trust from that first visit to know that the teacher is contacting them out of concern, with a desire to understand, problem solve, and communicate rather than to blame or complain.

Knowing a home situation can make a difference in how teachers interact with and support students. Kindergarten teacher Heather Tedford says "For teachers who don't do that, they don't actually realize where their students are coming from. Some of these teachers don't understand where these kids are coming from. That connection is really key" (Tedford, 2017, personal communication). This is especially true for children who come from households and neighborhoods different than the environments in which the teacher has spent her time. One of the most important steps a teacher can take in serving her students is to understand the ways in which that child looks at the world and makes meaning, and meeting with the family can help come to that understanding.

Relationships with families are often crucial not only to the child's well-being and health and success at school, but to the adults, who may well be struggling with issues that make it difficult to attend to their children as they would like. A relationship with their child's teacher and with other staff at the school can serve as a major support for the whole family.

> For many of the people we work with in our community, poverty is the biggest issue of diversity, and relationship is the most important thing to them. So, if we can connect with them and build relationships, which our kindergarten teachers do beautifully, that's our first line of defense. (Tracie McCarthy, 2017, personal communication)

Cautions

There are some obvious cautions and limitations to what is possible through home visits. Some families may be uncomfortable with a teacher coming into their home, for any number of reasons. Finding another place to meet in their community is an alternative; it still communicates the teacher's willingness to come to where the family is, especially for families that do not live in the neighborhood in which the school sits, and it begins the relationship between the child and her family and the teacher. The teacher can arrange with the family to meet in a location that is most comfortable for the family. When a child is homeless the relationship she has with her teacher becomes another potential anchor, and whatever the teacher can do to create a solid connection with her, and with her family will support a successful school experience, so a "home" visit can happen even with families who are homeless, meeting with the family in a location that is most comfortable to them.

Picnics or Before School Gatherings

Home visits may not be comfortable or practical for every teacher, but there are other ways to make connection with families before school begins. When I taught third grade in the north end of our city about one third of our students were bused up from the south end. They were mostly students of color (Seattle still tends to be much more segregated than its reputation would suggest), and most of them were living in relative poverty. They would take forty-five-minute bus rides to get to school each day, and it was difficult if not impossible for their families to be directly involved with the school, living at such a distance and dealing with the complex of working, child care, and public transportation. One of the steps I took was to hold a whole class picnic before the school year started at a park close by the school. We provided food, had adult and kid softball and soccer games, and spent time together in a very low stress context, getting to know each other.

We provided child care support for families with younger children, and rides to those families who did not have cars. We made sure to provide at least some food that everyone at the picnic could enjoy. It took a few hours to arrange (it would be quicker now, with computer connections), but it was well worth it.

This simple family picnic allowed several things to happen in a comfortable setting filled with good food, good fun, and a relaxed schedule. I had a chance to make connection with students who were new to me, and they had the opportunity to connect with me and with their new classmates. Their first sense of what this classroom was about was positive; there was a strong sense that what mattered most was the personal, and that all in the class were welcomed and valued. Watching them relax and have more and more fun as the day went on and then seeing their excitement and comfort level on the first day of school was further proof that our time together at the picnic had helped most of them move through at least some of their initial questions about this new classroom.

I also got to watch them be with each other, which helped me to get to know them as people. We know that children sitting at desks filling out assigned work are showing only one aspect of their total personalities; seeing them in other circumstances offers additional information about who they are and how they move through the world.

I had a chance to interact with their families, so I got to know more about where they came from, both by observing and by asking for the families to help me know what I should know about their children, as I described in the paragraphs about home visits. This also gave parents and families of the children in the class the opportunity to get to know each other and to develop connections with each other, which helped to build the classroom community.

Some knew each other from the neighborhood, or from having their children together in a previous grade, and some were meeting for the first time, and the connections among the parents and family members were an important part of our school year. They often came together to help with projects, on field trips, and to help children in the classroom, and they offered each other support as their children went through the ups and downs of the school year.

Finally, having the picnic near the school might have made the location a bit less threatening for families sending their children to school from a distance. They could picture the area and feel comfortable with the thought of their children there. They saw that we were willing to make the extra effort to help them to attend the picnic and hopefully saw that we would make the extra effort to take care of them during the school year.

Orientations at the School

Some teachers hold orientation sessions at the school, especially kindergarten teachers who are welcoming students and their families to school for the first time. Kindergarten teachers at Morrisonville Elementary hold orientations on two different days just before the opening of school. Two of the "K-team" talked about their orientation.

> It is a good way to set up a relationship. [...] We are going to work together to make this experience successful for your child. That whole child is going to be built right here, together. And if there are problems or issues we can figure this out together because now we've met you. So, it's not scary, school is not such a scary place. (Heather Tedford, 2017, personal communication)

Merri Jeanne Brennan (another of the K-team) continues.

> That's the initial piece that's needed, because parents need to feel that we are on their team and we're trying to create a healthy child; they have their trust in us right from the get-go. We feel by some point in the year that we really are a part of the family, they really do have that trust in us, but that comes from building that relationship, which takes a lot of time, and it's essential. (Brennan, 2017, personal communication)

The kindergarten team brings half their classes and their families on one day and the other half the next into the classroom so that the children can see the room they will be in, meet their classmates and teacher, get to play and be comfortable in this new setting. They see where they will sit, where to hang their coats and where the bathrooms are. All of those little things that make a huge difference in getting used to such a new experience. It also gives families and teachers to meet and start their relationship, as I described earlier.

Middle and High School

It is more challenging for teachers to make strong connections with all the families of the students they work with because there are so many more students (150, compared to 25), and because each student has several teachers rather than just one. I always sent letters home (my work at high school and middle school was before computers and email), outlining my basic goals and philosophy, inviting parent participation, and encouraging them to contact me if they had any questions or concerns. They were always welcome to come into the classroom to observe, and I invited them to come in to share knowledge or skills or experience related to what we were studying.

Some middle school and high school classes send newsletters home, these days via email (and hard copy for those households that do not have email), talking about the learning and projects they are engaged with in class. Depending on the class and time of year, this is a responsibility the students can handle, with the teacher including her own letter home as part of the newsletter. Others have exhibitions throughout the year where students share work they are doing, with families invited; some of these are during the day and some scheduled in the evenings in hopes of reaching as many families as possible.

Schools regularly schedule open houses during the first month of the school year so that families can come in the evening and walk through their student's schedule, spending a few minutes meeting with each teacher. That is an opportunity to literally hand materials that invite involvement and communication directly to family members (knowing that not all written material ever leaves the students' backpacks, lockers, or folders into which it was stuffed). There is rarely enough time to have in-depth conversations with families at these open houses, but it is an opportunity to say hello and to open the door for future meetings should that be desired.

I did spend time calling households when I taught middle and high school, giving myself permission to call a few each night so by the end of the first month of school I had contacted nearly every household. It was a significant investment of time and in some cases made a significant difference, especially when there were issues to discuss later in the year. There were students whose attendance was spotty, or who seemed particularly disengaged, and I found it useful to build on those first phone calls, to follow up with my concerns, and it was always appreciated by the families, who came to trust that I really was on their side, and more importantly, on their child's side.

Welcoming Students to School

Jamaal Bowman, principal at CASA Middle School in the Bronx, says it's all about relationships. He wants to make sure that students "feel loved from the moment they walk in the door, from a handshake to a hug, to a warm smile, to warm engagement." He is out front at the start of the school day, welcoming students into the building, making clear that he is very glad that they are a part of the school community. He gets to know the students and it helps him to get a read on what is happening in their lives and in the community. He might also connect with a family member who is dropping off his or her child, to check in with them briefly about how things are going, or to communicate something to them.

Many teachers make sure to welcome students coming into their room at the beginning of the day, either at the doorway, or during a transition period at the start of the day. They may have an open quiet play time or some sort of morning work at the start of the day to engage the students as they (the teachers) walk around the room checking in with students, or they might call each student up to speak with them, to hand in homework, to say good morning. Starting the day with this relationship-building time makes a significant difference for many students, including those whose days did not start out so well at home that morning. The teacher can ascertain whether the student had a good night's sleep, whether they have had breakfast, whether they need anything that will help get them ready to be at school. Checking in with students as they enter the room can often help to head off potential problems. If a teacher notices that a student is upset, or angry, or sad on the way into class she can respond to what she has noticed with whatever is appropriate; a high five, a hug, a kind word, a suggestion that the student might want to go get a drink and then come back to class, or she might get the rest of the class working on an assignment and spend some time with the student who may simply need to be heard for a couple of minutes.

There was a student I worked with who was volatile and who lived in an extremely challenging situation, and I could tell when he walked through the door how the night or morning had been for him. I would either get an enthusiastic high five from him or a stone face, promising an eruption in the near future. We worked out a routine where, if it was a stone face morning I would send him on an errand, either delivering attendance to the office, or something that gave him time to walk around the school a bit, to settle himself down before returning to the classroom. As the year went on he was able to let me know that he needed this walk and learned to ask for it. When he returned to class he was often ready to work, or to talk about what had happened, which he would do after I got his classmates started on their work.

When I taught in a middle school the principal asked all the teachers to stand at the doors of our classrooms between periods. There was grumbling, of course, since those precious few minutes enabled us to get ready for the next class, but her message was clear. We were to be at the door, able to see into the hallways. While we stood in those doorways we interacted with students as they flowed by, upstream or down towards their next classes. Saying hello, slapping high fives, offering a gentle reminder about the two minutes they had left to get to their seats.

As small an act as it is, it is an act of relationship. In the midst of hundreds of students passing by we are seeing individuals and connecting with them. We are connecting with the students as they enter, assessing quickly how they are doing, recognizing them and making clear that we are glad they are in school, in our classes. At a time when these young children are on the cusp of beginning their journeys as young adults, they are desperate for connections, for models, as Deborah Meier noted, and the simple act of reaching out to them is one response to that need, and as mentioned earlier, it helps us to gauge where our students are as they come into our classrooms, and what they might need.

Getting to Know Students as Learners and as People

When the year starts teachers and students really don't know each other, beyond whatever reputation has filtered through (what students have heard about particular teachers, or what teachers have heard about particular students or groups of students). It becomes crucial to spend time building community in the room. That is something that is practiced in many elementary classrooms.

> What was critical were the relationships that I could form with children, and that meant that I had to have time to be with kids, to talk to kids, to get to know them, who was unhappy, or when they were feeling successful, when one was left out or on

> the edges, when a kid didn't know what to do with all of their anger, when a kid was thriving at something, when groups were thriving or not thriving. Understanding the dynamics of the group also meant understanding the dynamics of the individuals. You don't build relationships with children without having room and time and energy for it. (Ruth Charney, 2018, personal communication)

This led her to develop structures in her classroom to offer her multiple opportunities to deepen relationships with her students, and to make sure they had the opportunity to develop relationships with each other. Morning meeting, one of the basic Responsive Classroom structures, came out of this recognition that there were classrooms in which the students did not even know the names of their classmates and had no relationship, or connection with them.

A room that is working at peak efficiency is a room in which all are working to support each other as learners, and as people. That does not just happen by accident; it happens because of many steps teachers take in guiding students to appreciate their role as both individuals and as members of a learning community, and that allows/enables the teacher to learn about the learners as individuals and as members of the group. When the group has come together as a learning community, everyone benefits. Students feel safer and more comfortable, more willing to take learning risks, more willing to reach out and help their neighbor. Students are more willing to be open about what they don't know when they feel they will not be teased about it, which means they will be more likely to get the help and support they need. Many of us in high school felt somewhat alone and alienated though we did not often admit it to anyone, and we assumed that everyone else had it more together than we did. Creating a space that helps students to find safety and connection is one of the greatest gifts you can offer them.

Having class discussions about how they want the room to function so that all can learn most effectively can be surprisingly effective, even with younger students. We can ask students to share what helps them to be most successful as learners and take that collective information as the basis for making decisions together about how the room will function. All are involved and responsible for determining their learning environment. The teacher is listening carefully, again learning from what the students share, but she also is demonstrating a real trust in the students as the room rules and decisions are made. This does not mean that anything goes, and the teacher has the final responsibility for what happens in the room, but how she manages that process is up to her and to the students. It is best to include some assessment pieces; how will the group know if things are working or whether the decision needs to be revisited. This gives everyone the message that decisions can be changed, that there is a responsibility to make sure folks are getting what they need as learners and community members, and that the goal and focus of the year is on learning.

Advisory and Parent Involvement

Class meetings and relationship building activities can happen at the secondary level as well. While there is not one way to approach having students get to know each other and to make strong connections, it is an important action to take. Consider that students are moving from an elementary setting where they are spending their whole day with one teacher and twenty to twenty-five classmates into a setting where they are moving through five or six different, disconnected classes, with five or six different sets of classmates. It is very easy to get lost, to feel "adrift," to use Deborah Meier's word, and whatever we can to help them feel more connected, to adults, to other students, the more engaged and supported they are likely to be. Many middle schools use some form of advisory, or homeroom to give students a sense of belonging and stability. The MET school, the flagship school of the Big Picture network started by Dennis Littky and Elliot Washor builds their program around what they call advisory. Littky quotes fellow educator George Wood talking about why advisory is so important:

> "[...] Advisory in one word is communication. It makes the school smaller. [...] Students know there is someone there for them, they are not getting lost among all the other students. [...] in advisory we don't talk at kids, we talk with kids." (Wood, quoted in Littky, 2004, 62)

Littky says that "setting up a system where students have **a consistent environment where they are able to truly connect with a small group of kids and one adult** (bold in original text) can radically change their entire schooling experience" (Littky, 2004, 62).

Advisories can play an important role in students feeling safe, in feeling connected, and in developing the ability to deal with problems. Here students talk about the benefits they experience from advisory.

> *Everyone in the school shares that bond that everyone has an advisor. So, from 6th grade to 12th grade, everyone shares that connection with one teacher, and I think that*

everyone throughout the day has opened up to someone. It gets you into the state of mind that school is not only about work, but that it is a place where teachers really know you and understand you. So, I think, as a school, having advisory connects everyone.
–eighth grade boy

When you have violence problems or drug problems or even academic problems or personal problems ... with your advisors and the things that the advisories provide do make you feel more close. ... It is a place where you can get stuff off your chest. And once you do, you rethink what you are doing and think, is this right? So that helps with your school work. (Shulkind and Foote, n.d. Italics in original)

Shulkind and Foote offer characteristics of an effective advisory:

- Strong advisory programs address issues of community.
- Strong advisories promote open communication.
- Strong advisors know and care about their advisees.
- Strong advisors closely supervise their advisees' academic progress.
- Strong advisors are problem solvers and advice givers.
- Students and advisors perceive that advisory directly improves academic performance.
- Students and advisors perceive that advisory functions as a community of learners.
(Shulkind and Foote, n.d.)

There are many ways to structure conversations within advisories, but it is important that there is intention and focus on building relationships, in establishing trust, and in helping students to develop the skills of listening and communicating with each other so that they can develop deeper relationships with peers and with their advisor.

Some teachers start the year with a survey of their students, asking them to share the ways they learn best, what they feel their learning strengths and challenges are, what helps them to be the best student they can be and what can get in the way, and what they want the teacher to know about them, so that she can be most useful to them. I know teachers who teach students about multiple intelligences and learning styles, to provide them with more information about the multiple ways that people learn. There have been times when I have done that and had real breakthroughs with students who had been convinced they were stupid, that they couldn't learn. They came to realize that even though they were not highly skilled at the traditional school approaches of reading and writing, they were intelligent in other areas such as hands-on learning, or working with others, or in artistic projects, for example. They began to appreciate their strengths and, when I made sure to offer assignments that gave them room to use those strengths they were able to perform at a high level, which did wonders for their confidence and self-image. It also helped others to see them differently.

I remember one middle school student who had never gotten a grade above a "C" in any of his classes, who made the most beautiful three-dimensional map of Washington State, much to the surprise of everyone else in the class (including me). It turns out he loved making models, and so this assignment, to create a three-dimensional map of the state was just right for him. He received a well-deserved "A" for the assignment and much respect from his classmates and others in the school as we displayed our maps in the library.

Another important aspect of community is to make sure that the room is welcoming to all students. Posters or artwork, quotes or other artifacts that represent high achievement from the cultures of the students in the room, and beyond, make clear that this room is open to the wider world, and that all cultures are welcome and valued.

This should also move beyond what is on the walls, to the curriculum. Principal Jamaal Bowman talks about it this way:

> Children seeing themselves in the curriculum so that the curriculum is culturally responsive, that's also a key piece. Oftentimes, especially for children of color the curriculum only talks about how they were dominated, colonized, imperialized. It doesn't talk about their cultures' contributions to the world and their achievements. (Bowman, 2018, personal communication)

He suggests ways that can happen:

> Making sure that there are positive representations of people of significance from all the cultures and ethnicities in the student body. When students see diverse representations that mirror the population of the school it makes clear that all belong in the school, all have the potential to do wonderful things, and that there is an expectation that all will be honored and celebrated. This can be done in so many different ways. The most obvious is to feature posters of prominent members of the various communities found in the school, and perhaps students can research and write summary bios of those featured on the walls. It can also work to coordinate with members of the school and surrounding community to feature notable figures from the various communities, again with students researching and telling their story. People from the community may not be so well known as those figures on full size posters, but they have the advantage of living in the town (or having lived in the town) and being (or having been) active in the local community. (Bowman, 2018, personal communication)

A deeper step in this move to recognize and honor the full diversity of the student body is to make sure the curriculum is a curriculum responsive to who is in the school. This often means going beyond the textbook and the state mandated curriculum, to include the voices and experiences of many more of the communities that make up the population of the United States, especially those cultures and communities connected to the children in the seats of the school.

Offering a curriculum that features the voices, accomplishments and stories of a wide range of cultures is important even in schools where the student body is not racially or ethnically diverse. All students (not just students of color) are more fully educated when they are exposed to and learn about the contributions of, and the histories of the many cultures that make up this country and world. Seeing posters of a diverse array of significant contributors to our society and studying the history and cultures of the full range of our people helps them to appreciate a more honest and complete understanding of the country's history. Otherwise, we are depriving them of knowledge and understanding that they need to be informed, educated citizens of the world.

Claire Oglesby, who taught for more than forty years in an elementary school in Vermont made a point to "study" the world in her classroom. She said that since Vermont was the whitest state in the union she had an even greater responsibility to help her students to appreciate and value diversity of all sorts, and to move past ignorance and stereotypes. The film *The World in Claire's Classroom* offers a snapshot of a year in which she helps her young students to learn about the world, to a surprising depth.

When working with elementary students, we have more time to spend getting to know them since there are fewer of them and we are together for most of the school day, so I invite them to share more of their out of school lives with each other. That can be through class meetings, where we share what we do for chores, favorite movies or music, sports, or activities. They have writing assignments that ask them to describe a favorite place so that we appreciate what it is like to be in that place (which also serves a language arts objective), or their favorite meal, or to tell a time they did something that was a little scary or challenging.

I also give them the assignment to document a typical day. When I first offered this assignment, it was before the internet and cell phones, so we gave each student a bargain basement 35 mm camera (which came through a grant I wrote) and sent them off to document important aspects of their lives. They decided what to include, what to say about the photos they included, and how to present it to the rest of us. These days, given the available media, it is probably not necessary to write a grant to buy cameras, though of course it will not hurt to have a few on hand in case someone does not have a cell phone or other device.

The point of these assignments (and I offer this only as one example; there are thousands of them) is to have students (and teachers, who do this as well) get to share a bit more of who they are, and what matters to them with the learning community. The primary focus of the assignment is building community and having each child feel more fully accepted and appreciated as a part of the class, but it also meets many learning objectives in language arts and in social studies and can serve as the basis for further assignments based on what the students have shared.

Getting to know the community the students come from is important as well. Teacher Educator Maria Timmons Flores talks about a community project carried out in Bellingham WA that helps those working with students from migrant families to learn more about the students and their families:

> They (students from migrant worker families) worked with one of their bilingual teachers to create a video project. [...] She put out a box and said, what would you tell your teachers if you felt safe telling them? And then she and this other migrant advocate sent cameras home with the kids to take pictures of their lives. That was really transformative for the students, to share these things, anonymously, at first, but then to have conversations about what to include and how they were going to share them and sequence them and who they wanted to show it to. The first time they showed it the students were not present, but they gave permission to show it to their teachers. And it made a dramatic shift. The teachers came away and said, "oh my god, all this time I've been asking them why they didn't bring their homework to school, and now it's shifted to, how are you, I notice your homework is not here, what's going on and how can we make this happen? What can I do to support you to get that learning done?" So, it really did make a shift and the kids noticed that and it was really empowering for them.
>
> That team of the ELL educator, and the migrant advocate put out a notice asking who would like to learn more about Mextico culture, migrant culture and students. They expected a handful and they had sixty teachers in their district who responded. They brought parents in to talk about different themes, from their language and culture, to their history and traditions, what brought them here, to some of the arts and crafts from that part of the world. (Maria Timmons Flores, 2016, personal communication)

When families are feeling more welcomed and heard, when students are feeling more understood and supported, there is more likely to be a healthy relationship between home and school, geared towards helping the children be successful.

There are other opportunities to communicate respect and trust to students. Some teachers do not require students to ask permission to go to the rest room. They tell the students that they (the class) have discussed when it is a good time to go and leave it to the students to be responsible about making the choice without needing permission. The same with getting a drink; Are you thirsty? Is this a good time to get a drink (you won't be missing instructions for the assignment)? Then go get a drink; you don't need to ask. These practices communicate to the students that we trust them to make good decisions, for themselves and for the group.

Being Available, Being Accessible, and Reaching Out

Being available at lunch, after school, or whenever students need to talk is another step that helps build relationships. It began for me during my first year of teaching high school when I realized that eating in the teachers' lunch room was making me sick. It wasn't only the air, though at the time there was smoking allowed. It was the negative energy that at least a few of the teachers felt comfortable spewing. I know that some of it was blowing off frustration and other emotions that had built up during the morning so that they could return in a more balanced state for the afternoon, but some of it was the venom of teachers who had maybe loved teaching at one time but clearly did not love it any longer. Their nastiness was poisonous and made our otherwise blissful twenty-five minutes of lunch very uncomfortable.

I started eating in my room, alone or with a few colleagues. On occasion a student might stop by to talk and over time that became a more regular routine for at least a few students, another opportunity to find connection. We often talked of mundane matters (how about those Mariners), but at times there were more serious and personal issues that came up, and we had some time to talk them through.

Lunchtime is also a very important time in elementary school. It's obviously different than the high school experience; the children are younger, they are with their teachers all day rather than shifting to a new class and teacher every period, and there are usually no more than thirty in a classroom (often fewer), so it is possible to develop relationships with the students. Even with that, much of the learning time is structured such that the focus is on the assignment, and the teacher's time is divided among those twenty-five to thirty students so that no one gets exclusive, focused time. That can change at lunch.

One school I taught at had no lunchroom, so we ate in the classroom. The lunches were prepared at a central district location and delivered to the school, and we then picked them up and ate as a class before recess. It was a relatively relaxed time and the students would play games and have conversations and enjoy music that one of them would bring to class. It was a time for us to regroup and to enjoy being together. It was also, at times a chance to have extended conversations with students who needed that time to talk, and frequently one would stay in during recess because they needed/wanted that time.

I want to be clear: teachers do need their all too short lunch periods to rest and recover a bit, though mostly what happens is that they run around making phone calls, copies, and attending to the many details that lead to a successful afternoon while attempting to eat at least part of what they brought for lunch. I was not in the daily habit of giving up every lunch recess period, but made sure that once or twice a week I made that option available. Having time for the class to spend relaxed stretches of time together, and for teachers and students to connect on a person to person level makes a significant difference in the school experience teachers and students can have.

Lunch With Tracie

Another lunch time strategy employed by the teachers and school psychologist at Morrisonville Elementary resulted in most all K-3 students having lunch with "Miss Tracie" at some point during the semester. Tracie, the school psychologist, started to have lunch with a few students from the kindergarten through third grade classes along with a student or two on the autistic spectrum, hoping that lunching with others in a small group would help the students on the spectrum to acquire some comfort and social skills through the interactions.

The K-3 students loved their time with Tracie, and soon her lunch "dance card" was full, which was wonderful in that the students got to spend some quality time with a caring and skilled adult, but also because they were developing a deeper relationship with a person they might well be talking to if they had problems or issues to work out. The lunch routine also helped Tracie to make deeper connection with families.

"The parents realize this as well because I'll get many calls, oh Miss Tracie, so and so comes to see you at lunch [...] and they're not sleeping so well, they're not eating so well [...] and I they don't know exactly what I do [...]" (Tracie McCarthy, 2017, personal communication).

Attending Events

I know many teachers who make a point of attending as many student-involved events as possible. It means a great deal to the students that they are there, and it is another opportunity to build relationship with parents who attend. They see you are taking the time to support their children, and there can be a lot of time to talk during soccer games. I saw many sports events, plays, musical performances, and art shows, again showing to students that I cared about them, was interested in what they were doing, and was going to support them.

This can also turn around relationships in the classroom. I was teaching ninth grade world history and had a couple of young men who were not engaged with the material, with their classmates or with me. They were baseball players and that's all that mattered. I had a couple of unproductive meetings with them, and we seemed destined to have an uncomfortable semester together. I went to a couple of their baseball games; I also taught other students who played on the team, so I wasn't going just to see the two in my history class. We started talking baseball around the edges of the history class (I played when I was younger) and began to develop a relationship. I won't say that they became passionate world history students, but they did begin to engage with me and with the class. They cared that I cared about what mattered to them.

Physical Health

Physical health is one of the key determinants of overall health, and while there are limits to what we can control outside of school there are definite things we can do inside.

There are basic ways in which we can work with other community agencies and institutions in addition to resources within the school community to support the physical health and well-being of our students, and it is, as they say, not rocket science. First off, schools and community, working together, can provide basic health checks and care at the schools. Some of this already happens, with schools doing basic health screenings, and many schools in wealthier districts have full time nurses in the schools. Community health clinics can be located at or adjacent to the schools so that children can get the care they need, and it also makes it easier for families to get care as well, saving them an extra trip to clinics located elsewhere in the city or town. Dental facilities can also be a part of this health cluster, again serving both children and their families in a centrally located complex.

But health, as we have seen is much more than regular health checkups and prompt treatment, when needed, though that's a great place to start.

Food and Nutrition

Food is an essential part of physical health, and while most schools offer breakfasts and lunches, the quality and appeal of what's offered have given rise to many generations of jokes and nightmares. The quality is often low because the budget schools have for feeding our children is low, but if we are committed to the health of our children we can make it a priority to provide nutritious and tasty food for both breakfast and lunch. As things are now, we know there are significant inequalities in what students are getting, both at home and at school.

Getting healthy, nutritious food to the children is a crucial and relatively inexpensive action we can take. It is definitely much cheaper than the cost of dealing with the many illnesses and health conditions arising from poor nutrition.

> In America, one out of every three kids is overweight or obese, and at-risk for Type 2 Diabetes. This generation of children is predicted to have shorter life expectancies than their parents, primarily due to their diets. [...] Ensuring kids have access to healthy, fresh school food is a crucial part of the solution.
>
> More than 30 million children eat school lunch every day, and over 70% (22 million) of these kids come from impoverished households. The eating habits and food values they learn in childhood will follow them for the rest of their lives. So, for now, while our kids are still young, and we're still filling their lunch trays, we have an opportunity to shape the future. When we make sure that our children's meals are cooked with real food, instead of food additives and chemicals, we set them up for a lifetime of healthy eating habits that help them grow, thrive, and achieve. (Miller, 2016)

There are an increasing number of school programs that are bringing healthier options to children in schools. Some of them are doing it in collaboration with local farms, offering farm to table options. The Communities That Care program for Franklin County/North Quabbin (Massachusetts) recently completed a study of school lunch programs for all districts within their region and brought the heads of food service together to share what each was doing, to learn from each other about how they can both provide healthier alternatives to all students and how they can entice their students to take advantage of those healthier alternatives. More schools are offering salad bars, providing nutritional information and education to students about healthy eating, shopping, and cooking, and creating gardens on school grounds. When the students grow food and then eat what they grow they make a meaningful connection between where their food comes from, what it offers them by way of health benefits, and tends to make them more open to eating that food. I talk more about this program in the next chapter.

Connecting Schools With Farms

There has been an increasing interest in connecting schools with local farms, both for its educational value, with students learning where their food comes from and how to grow it, and for the nutritional benefit of having fresh, organic vegetables and fruit in their cafeterias. One such connection is happening on Bainbridge Island, Washington, located just across Puget Sound from Seattle. Bainbridge Island was home to hundreds of Japanese Americans in the first decades of the twentieth century, and after years of working and improving the rocky soil of that island they established profitable strawberry farms. They would bring their produce into Seattle to sell at the Pike Place Market. That is until they were all rounded up and incarcerated in internment camps during World War II. Most of the community returned to the island after the war and resumed farming.

Jon Garfunkel and Ed Mikel started the group Educulture on Bainbridge Island with the goal of connecting "the science, the culture, the people, the history, the food—into a living, hands-on curriculum that reaches deep into the schools and into the community at large" (Reinke, 2018). The group started working with one school on the island in 2006 and has since expanded to working with several elementary and middle schools, matching schools with local farms closest to their school.

Students from the schools have made connections with local farmers, developing relationships that have led to students learning much more about what it means to farm, and to farm organically. They have gone out to work in the fields and farmers have come into the schools, an exchange that has led to more understanding and appreciation for all concerned, and the schools are serving local, organic food grown on the farms they have come to know.

The Chicago Public Schools is an example of a school district taking steps to take on the challenges of providing nutritious meals, and a program supporting children to eat healthy. They put out this announcement at the start of the 2017–2018 school year:

> Chicago Public Schools (CPS) will provide free breakfast and lunch to all CPS students, regardless of their economic eligibility, for the first time beginning this school year due to the district's expansion of the Community Eligibility Provision (CEP).
>
> This program will allow all CPS students to focus on their studies without being distracted by hunger or worry about the stigma of free or reduced lunch," said Barbara Byrd-Bennett, Chief Executive Officer of CPS. Formerly known as the Community Eligibility Option (CEO), the Community Eligibility Provision (CEP) of the Healthy, Hunger-Free Kids Act of 2010, allows qualifying high-need school districts to offer free breakfast and lunch to all students, providing the nutrition and energy children need to be healthy and ready to learn. (CPS Nutrition Support Services)

In the 2010–11 school year, CPS adopted new nutrition standards that included serving more fruit and vegetables, and more whole grains, limiting less healthy foods such as fries, nachos, doughnuts and pastries, and sugary breakfast cereals. They have also taken other steps to improve the nutrition of their students:

- **Scratch Cooking.** Thanks to recent facility upgrades, more schools have the equipment and training to cook fresh meals from scratch.
- **Farm to school.** CPS has a robust farm to school program that provides students with tasty, nutritious produce while supporting local farmers and communities. CPS has purchased more than $4.2 million in produce from regional farmers over the past three school years.
- **Antibiotic-free chicken.** CPS sources and regularly serves chicken raised without the use of antibiotics from a local farm.
- **Breakfast in the classroom.** This initiative offers all elementary students a free breakfast when they arrive at school. An extensive body of research shows that breakfast consumption positively influences students' cognitive function, focus, attention and emotional well-being.
- **Healthy Snack and Beverage Policy.** This recently adopted policy establishes nutrition standards for food available to students outside the school lunch program, including a la carte items sold in the cafeteria, vending machines, fundraisers and school stores.
- **Community Eligibility.** Through the Community Eligibility Provision of the Healthy, Hunger-Free Kids Act, CPS is able to provide

> free breakfast and lunch to all CPS students, removing the red tape and stigma associated with free and reduced price meals. (School Food Policy, n.d.)

I've quoted from their material at length to offer the breadth of their approach to helping their children move towards a healthy approach to nutrition, from farm to table and beyond. It is complex. In these tight times people notice the costs of such a program, and federal subsidies for meals are so small that it is a particular challenge, but when you measure those costs against what it costs to address the diseases and conditions that arise out of unhealthy eating, ranging from obesity to high blood pressure to heart attacks and strokes, the money spent up front on helping children to live healthy and to be ready and able to learn is a bargain, not to mention that we are talking about our children, and having them live healthy lives is, to quote some ad or another, priceless.

Farm to school programs are increasing across the country.

> Today, the USDA released new data from its 2015 Farm to School Census and [...] farm to school activities have grown from a handful of schools in the late 1990s to reaching 23.6 million students nationwide. According to the data, 5,254 school districts—a total of 42,587 schools across all 50 states and Washington D. C.—participate in farm to school activities, including serving local food in the cafeteria, holding taste tests and taking students on field trips to farms and orchards. (Talis, 2016)

The National Farm to Schools Network has extensive resources to help interested districts and communities get started in making this transition. They have produced a brochure to help make this happen; you can find it at http://www.farmtoschool.org/Resources/Getting%20Started%20with%20Farm%20to%20School.pdf.

Snacks

Another piece of the food picture is in-class snacks. Most every school and classroom has a snack policy, and many students bring snacks from home, the quality of which runs from admirable to appalling. Recognizing that what children bring to school is a reflection of a complex mix of economics, the availability of nutritious food in neighborhoods, time to shop, awareness of what healthy eating looks like, cultural values and practices, and more, many teachers keep snacks on hand. The costs of providing the snacks comes out of the teachers' already thin pockets, so what they can afford to offer is less than what they wish they could offer. This is another area that lends itself to connecting with community resources, from orchards and farms to local supermarkets, farmers' markets, and the like. The farm to school network can be of use here as well.

Backpack Programs

The concerns about food at school are very real, as are concerns about the food the children don't get to eat when school is closed over weekends, vacations, or through the summer. As marginal as the food may be at school, it is something, which is more than some children get at home.

Backpack programs have become a more regular presence in many of our schools located in communities that are struggling financially. Schools have recognized that for many of our students living in severe poverty, the meals they get at school are the only meals they may eat. When there is no school, over weekends or school vacations, they worry that these students may not have anything to eat, so they have started to send backpacks home with food for those no-school days. The budget for these programs is small so the food that is sent home tends to be processed food and of low nutritional value, but it is certainly better than nothing, and hopefully it is a start towards improving the quality of food sent home.

The Greenfield Public Schools has begun a summer program that will offer free breakfast and lunch to children over the summer. This is the announcement they have posted on their web site:

> Starting Monday, June 25th, 2018, free meals to children and youth 18 and under will be available, Monday through Friday, June 25th–August 17th, as well as Saturdays, July 1st–August 12th.

They are offering the meals at a variety of locations around town, including at sites of low-income housing, and are offering raffle tickets for a free bicycle for students who come to get breakfast as an added inducement for students to take part in the program. It is an example of a district recognizing that the needs of the students don't stop when the school year ends and that the school can continue to serve them through the summer.

Cooking Classes

There are school programs, usually held after school, to teach children how to cook simple, nutritious meals, and given the concern about obesity and the number of children who are not eating nutritious foods, that number is spreading. Schools have connected with local restaurants, with food coops, local farms, and others to bring an awareness of what it means to eat in a healthy way, and how to shop for and cook/prepare nutritious meals. There are grants available to support such programs, and often local restaurants or stores are willing to donate time and materials to the effort. Once more, the farm to school network can help to make this happen.

An extension of this is to offer classes to families, and while this is even more complicated, given the restrictions most family have on time and resources, holding cooking classes in community centers, in neighborhood centers, or in facilities connected to local religious institutions can help families to learn how to eat healthier.

Just Roots

Jay Lord is a former teacher, one of the creators of Responsive Classroom, and one of the founders of Just Roots, an organization dedicated to linking farming and education. He talked about one of the programs that Just Roots ran in a local elementary school in Greenfield, Massachusetts.

> We set up gardens, we set up all kinds of stuff and they totally bought in. They had compost and they wanted to get chickens and they had festivals and they wanted to get gardens. We set up a tomato table where all the tomatoes had been made into food and the parents would come and try them. We had snack markets there and later we made soups in the classroom, which they loved, and they had them for their lunches [...]
>
> We would come in every Friday in the fall [...] We had three stations. The first station was, the students would have to try something new; it was something raw. We brought in all kinds of weird stuff, but it was all local. And then we would involve them in research about who likes what, and then they'd take their snack away from a big table that had lots of choices. It was incredible. They loved it, and the kids, after three years they'd try anything. (Lord, personal conversation, 2018)

Creating Gardens at School

Creating gardens at the school is a wonderful way for children to become more familiar with where their food comes from, to become acquainted with what fresh food looks like and tastes like, and to learn to cook with it to prepare nutritious meals.

Researchers and teachers have noted numerous benefits to starting a garden at school. Among them:

- Increased consumption of fruits and vegetables
- Improvement in attitudes towards fruits and vegetables
- Improvement in science achievement scores
- Improvement in social skills and behaviors
- Improvement in environmental attitudes and instillation of respect for nature
- Positive impact on student achievement and behavior (Kidsgardening.org, n.d.)

There are several sites on the internet offering advice about how to plan and begin a garden: all of them advise to take time to be clear about your goals and resources, to have a large vision but to begin small so that you can have success, knowing you can build on that. The available resources or assets in each community are unique to that community, so who is available to support this effort will vary, and that is where some of your early steps would focus; what expertise, person power, financial resources, and time are available to help. In what ways will children be involved in working in/with the garden, and how will their work in the garden be incorporated into the classroom and lunchroom.

There may well be gardeners in the school or surrounding community who would be willing to help. There may well be suppliers, farmers, coops or others who would donate necessary materials. School work parties might be an option for setting up the growing plots. There is not one way to do this; what is clear is that the potential for benefit for the students is real and worth exploring.

Recess and PE

There is extensive research supporting the need of children to move, to be physically active every day. What we have seen happening at schools is that they are moving away from moving; recess has been cut back as has PE, crowded out by test preparation. When I taught at elementary grades there was recess in the morning, recess at lunch, and a brief recess in the afternoon. There were also gym classes several days each week. That schedule is rare these days.

Many of the articles and papers about recess emphasize that children will be more effective learners if they get to move, and so they advocate for recess so that students get better grades, but more importantly, students need to move to be healthy.

Recess is a "crucial and necessary component of a child's development. Recess helps students develop communication skills, such as cooperation and sharing, and helps counteract the time they spend sitting in class." (Seaman, 2012)

The American Academy of Pediatrics put out a policy statement on recess:

> Recess represents an essential, planned respite from rigorous cognitive tasks. It affords a time to rest, play, imagine, think, move, and socialize. After recess, for children, or after a corresponding break time for adolescents, students are more attentive and better able to perform cognitively. In addition, recess helps young children to develop social skills that are otherwise not acquired in the more structured classroom environment …
>
> Recess promotes social and emotional learning and development for children by offering them a time to engage in peer interactions in which they practice and role play essential social skills. This type of activity, under adult supervision, extends teaching in the classroom to augment the school's social climate. Through play at recess, children learn valuable communication skills, including negotiation, cooperation, sharing, and problem solving as well as coping skills, such as perseverance and self-control. These skills become fundamental, lifelong personal tools. Recess offers a child a necessary, socially structured means for managing stress. By adapting and adjusting to the complex school environment, children augment and extend their cognitive development in the classroom. (Council on Health, 2013)

The Pediatricians also make the point that recess is not the same as P.E.; each has its own function and purpose, and one should not be substituted for the other. The focus in P.E. is on developing particular developmentally appropriate motor skills and is taught in structured, sequenced lessons. Recess is most valuable when it is unstructured (though supervised), when children have the freedom to make choices of whether to and how to interact with their peers.

Teaching Children to Play

One of the interesting challenges around recess is the number of children who do not know how to play. Many children seem to have little experience with unstructured play and so recess is a stressful situation for them. Ruth Charney said that their educational team developed what they called "structured play" as part of their program to help teach children how to play.

> We began at recess. It would turn into kids lolling around doing nothing, or a lot of aggression, or games that were all about power, so structured play and structured

> recess were important. The faculty went to recess with the students and played with them, helping them learn how to play, how to win, to lose, to negotiate, and how to have fun without hurting others. It was an important part of their curriculum. (Charney, 2018, personal communication)

I had to teach my third graders how to play because so many of them were kept inside by their families after school because of a fear of violence. Many of them did not know their neighbors (because they were bused to schools across town), so they spent the afternoons alone, in front of screens. I regularly went outside with them and played a variety of games, both teaching the rules and helping them learn to play together in ways that they all enjoyed. It was a teaching opportunity for many different aspects of their social emotional learning, and it was an opportunity for some students more physically "intelligent" than others to succeed in ways that they did not necessarily succeed in reading or math. Playing together at recess, and at other times helped us to develop as a learning community.

Opportunity to Learn and Grow

Schools help children to open and expand their world. Many of our children, especially those living in isolated rural communities, in inner city communities, or in severe poverty in any setting live in very narrow, circumscribed worlds. They do not have the resources or options to move out into the larger world. Professor Vincent Carey marvels at what schools can offer their students:

> Schools, healthy schools, provide access to culture to all their students. A healthy school and a healthy community. There are kids who go on annual elementary field trips, who get access to places, experiences, music, art, history, museums, that their parents, for a variety of reasons would never be able to provide them. They would never be able to get access to that one inspiring field trip, one enjoyable field trip … It is about culture, it is about access, it is about health, the well-being of students. (Carey, 2017, personal communication)

Schools offer students the opportunity to meet and learn with others, from within their neighborhoods and outside of them. Schools are places in which students can learn about their own neighborhoods and town through place-based education, guided and supported studies of their own towns and environment, where they can further their understanding of how and why systems intersect and why those systems have an impact on their lives. And they come to learn the ways in which people have worked for justice, have worked for change that made lives better for people.

Gary Thomsen, an extraordinary teacher who engaged his students in learning projects that broadened his students' sense of possibilities made that one of the central objectives of his curriculum. His students biked across country, retracing the route and collecting data about Negro League baseball players barnstorming across Canada, data they donated to the Negro League Baseball Museum in Kansas City (Selwyn, 2010). He also took students across country on roller blades, carrying a message about environmental awareness, and had still others research and then share the stories of immigrant communities living within their neighborhoods in Seattle. I asked Thomsen how he chose his projects and what his objectives were;

> A lot of kids that I see have two issues. Number one, they don't tend to think big. When I ask them what they want to do, they can't tell me. And two, most of them haven't had much success in their lives, so consequently they don't really think these projects are going to happen, they don't believe that they can collectively pull it off. So, in general, the goal of these projects is to give kids a sense of confidence and self-fulfillment while teaching them transferable skills that will help them throughout their lives. (Selwyn, 2010, 102)

All of our projects, big or small, involve a set of steps, and have to meet four criteria:

> Is the project relevant and can it be clearly defined?
> Does it have the potential to benefit the students after they leave high school/college?
> Does it benefit the community, local or national?
> Does it benefit the school/district?
> (Selwyn, 2010, 105)

Thomsen was working with a population that was mostly students of color, many of them from immigrant communities, and he was teaching them communication skills, computer skills, and research skills that would be essential and valuable to them no matter what path they took following school. Experiential learning provides the context for learning and practicing these skills because they must use them to complete the project; it is not just theoretical or intellectual learning going on here.

Gary also noted that traveling was very important, as many of his students had never really been out of their neighborhoods, some never more than two or three blocks from their home, and he wanted to broaden their sense of what was possible, and to have them experience the world.

Democratic Education, Internships, and Individualized Instruction

Summerhill is probably the most well-known of the schools organized around democratic principles. The school was founded by A. S. Neill in 1921, in England, and the guiding vision was (and remains) that students learn to be responsible, critical thinkers by having the freedom, opportunity and support to make important decisions that affect their own lives. They make decisions about what classes to take and whether to attend or not, and they meet as a community, with each person having one vote, from youngest child to the teachers and administrators in deciding policies and resolving issues. There is a fundamental trust that children will learn to make responsible decisions on their own behalf and on behalf of the community when they trust that they are taken seriously and not pressured to simply please adults. The school is still in existence, still adhering to its founding principles, and still successful.

There are many examples of democratic schools around the country, and they are "democratic" to a greater or lesser extent. What they have in common is that they trust the students to develop into responsible and informed decision makers when they have the opportunity to learn and to practice, and that the best preparation for being responsible adults is to be given responsibility and opportunity to be responsible citizens at a young age. There is an appreciation and recognition that there needs to be guidance and support for the students as they learn, grow, and mature into responsible decision makers, and that is one of the guiding missions of the school.

The MET school in Providence, Rhode Island is an example of a school that emphasizes decision making, critical thinking, and the right and necessity of students directing their own learning. The school offers each student the opportunity to engage in an intense internship with someone in the community in the area they want to explore. The MET is a public school, so the students are still responsible for meeting state requirements in a range of subject areas, but they study those areas, learn the required material as it relates to their chosen field of focus. The underlying assumption here is that students will bring much more energy, focus, and persistence to their studies if they care about what they are learning.

The results at the MET are proof that this approach serves the students well. Their graduation rate is above the state average, their dropout rates are below the state average, and they have now expanded their model to more than sixty schools around the country.

One of the keys to what makes the Met school work is that the students remain committed to the whole school learning community even as they are pursuing their individual passions. They take part in advisory, which is a key element to the program; they are with the same group of students and teacher/advisor for four years and support each other as learners. They also participate in all-school meetings and learn to balance their individual agenda with the needs and agenda of the whole school.

While most schools are not so heavily focused on their commitment to democracy, it is still very possible to offer students experience with decision making and community building within a more traditional structure. Here are a couple of steps that some teachers have taken that provide their students with the opportunity for real democratic engagement, and that demonstrate to students a sense of respect and trust.

First, many teachers engage students in developing the rules, norms, and practices of the classroom, as I mentioned earlier in the chapter. It is the students' classroom too and having them as active participants in deciding how the room should operate is a step towards creating democratic citizens and having each class member feel a part of the community. Having said that, it is the teacher's role to make sure that every voice is heard during discussion.

Second, there are many assignments that can allow students to pursue individual areas of interest that still meet the learning objectives of the teacher. For example, let's say that students are learning about persuasive writing. Having students write a persuasive piece on a topic that matters to them does not detract from the fundamental writing skills that are being taught, and will produce more honest, passionate, and carefully done work if the student really cares about what she is writing, and especially if what she writes will be sent to an authentic audience, someone who is relevant to her topic.

The same principle applies when teaching various research skills; why not give students room to learn and to demonstrate their learning through researching what matters to them? The same skills, the same depth of understanding would apply, but the students would bring more to the assignment and the students would be in position to help each other to learn since they were researching different topics.

Exhibitions are another variation on this theme, of having students research and put together presentations that demonstrate learning in whatever ways will most help them to communicate what they have found. The public format of their sharing means that their classmates will learn from them, both content and by how they have chosen to share their learning, and for some students, being able to choose how to present their work allows their creativity to show through. A public presentation also raises the stakes so that the students put more thought, care, and attention into their research and preparation. It is also an opportunity to invite parents and family members to be present at the exhibitions, furthering and deepening the connection between home and school.

Learning to Learn

There is no greater gift or tool we can offer our students, beyond our unconditional love, support and belief in them than in helping them to learn how to learn, to think critically, and to take responsibility for finding what they want to know.

Part of students learning to learn is helping them to break the chains of the negative messages they have heard all their lives about what they can't do, about how bad they are, or whatever the particular message happens to be. Milwaukee educator and artist Azeeza Islam focuses on helping her students to redefine themselves in terms of their gifts, and in their possibilities.

She calls her approach "master thyself," and gives her students

> [...] tools and support during the school year that ought to apply to their lives, whether at home or when they are out in public or wherever. I hold them responsible but then I also model it. I don't say one thing to them and then do another. I have to be consistent and be patient as well as consistent with the information I give to them on a regular basis.
>
> I'm sure for some people it's going to take hearing something once, and for others one thousand times. Some people may take more, so I have to always come back to them in the same way, each and every time to remind them. Because the way that I see them, I'm changing a lot of information. The children are coming into my classroom between the ages of four and maybe twelve. Those children are hearing the dialogue that they have in their head, they have been hearing that dialogue for all of those years. That talk is negative, about what they can't do, or how bad they are. If they get me for one year, I'm changing all the information that they've been getting thus far and trying to get them something different. Sometimes that's going to take a while ... I even found myself, even on the last day of school reminding them of some of the things I taught them on the first day of school. And to me that's ok. I know that some lose patience after they have said these things a few times, but that's not what children need. (Islam, 2018, personal communication)

Students can be introduced to and offered the opportunity to practice the fundamental skills of research, or inquiry, of asking real questions about things that matter to them and then pursuing those questions to their own satisfaction. The steps of inquiry, which I have written about in Following the Threads (Selwyn, 2010), are not complicated, but they take time, practice, and persistence, and most students will stay with those steps only if they truly care about what they are researching. Otherwise, it's just an empty exercise that they will complete for a grade, and then forget like a bad dream.

What is key to this approach of helping students learn how to learn is to not mistake the final product as the essential value of the assignment. It is about offering students the opportunity to research something they care about, to engage with the process of inquiry, and to learn from the experience, reflecting on what worked well and what they could do differently the next time. If we are most committed to having students come away from their learning experiences with skills, knowledge, and a sense of confidence that this is a process they will be able to use for the rest of their lives then our focus should be on what will help them to develop those skills and that confidence.

I worked with a student in a second/third grade classroom who panicked when given the assignment to create an imaginary island. All he had to do as a first step was to draw the outline of the island. Then he would create a map of the island followed by descriptions of one or two places on the island. The finale would be some sort of short story or play that took place in one of those places he had described. J. was afraid to draw the island because he was afraid he would get it wrong. I reasoned with him that since he was the only person who had seen this island, no one could tell him he was wrong, but that did not convince him to go ahead. After some time, I put a dot on his paper and handed him an imaginary spy glass. He could look through the spy glass, which enlarged the island so that only he could see the details. This allowed him to move forward a bit, and he eventually drew an island map that looked a whole lot like Skull Island, from Peter Pan, which was just fine. He got to engage in the assignment, learning about maps, about descriptions, and about writing stories, which was my agenda.

What was most concerning was that this eight-year old was already terrified of making a mistake, of suffering the slash of the red pen. He had suffered an assault that had left him wounded, and less likely and able to learn and grow. What are we doing to our children? And it's not only our young children who struggle with the consequences of such attacks.

I have taught with the Puget Sound Writing Project, the Seattle branch of the National Writing Project, for nearly twenty years and there are many teachers who have been wounded as writers by well-meaning teachers in their past who corrected them into writing paralysis, and who are now, many years later, trying to recover some degree of confidence and joy in the writing process. These are successful teachers and many of them teach writing to young people. They talk of having been taught, as J. was, to be afraid of making mistakes, of being so worried about misspelling a word or other minor error that they gave up trying to do anything beyond the minimum. They "learned" to write safe, boring, risk free sentences with words they could spell, even if they had other things to say and other ways to say it. They had been taught to avoid risk and the possibility of mistake at all costs and lost themselves as writers.

When I think of the damage done to these essentially successful students, college graduates and teachers, I shudder to think of what we have done to students who do not make it through to the end of the educational assembly line, the students who drop out, flame out, who are shoved out, who are labeled as failures at an early age and never move past that label.

Our purpose as educators is to help our students to grow into the healthiest, ablest people they can be, and to support them to develop the skills, knowledge, and approaches that will help them to sustain that health and well-being. We have the responsibility to create a safe learning space and community in which risk taking is encouraged, where there is an opportunity to learn, and that trying something new is celebrated as an attempt to learn a new step.

I also want to remind us that these steps are part of a much larger picture that is informed by what I've presented throughout the book. The actions I have suggested in this chapter can and will help our students to be healthier, and perhaps their grades will improve, but they are a small part of what must change if we want our children, our society, and our democracy to be healthier. Making sure there are healthy snacks on hand is important, especially for children who are coming to school hungry, but our larger work is to make sure they are not coming to school hungry. I'm not minimizing the importance of school-based actions but urging us to also keep in mind that it can't stop at the school level, but must move into the community and beyond, which I'll address in the next chapter.

References

Bowman, J. (2018). Personal communication.

Brennan, M. J. (2017). Personal communication.

Carey, V. (2017). Personal communication.

Charney, R. (2018). Personal communication

Council on Health 2013
Chicago Public Schools Nutrition Services. https://cps.edu/About_CPS/Departments/Pages/FoodServices.aspx
Flores, Maria Timmons. (2016). Personal communication
Islam, A. (2018). Personal communication.
Kidsgardening. (n.d.). Retrieved from Kidsgardening.org
Littky, D. (2004). Big picture: Education is everyone's business. Alexandria, VA: ASCD
Lord, J. (2018). Personal communication
McCarthy, T. (2017). Personal communication
Meier, D. (2002). In schools we trust: Creating communities of learning in an era of testing and standardization. Boston: Beacon.
Miller, E. (2016, October 11). Kids need #realschoolfood—and farm-to-school is making it happen. National Farm to School Network. Retrieved from http://www.farmtoschool.org/news-and-articles/tag/Healthier_Lunches/
Reinke, V. (2018, Summer). Growth experience: Educulture honors yesterday and teaches for tomorrow. Bainbridge Island Magazine, Issue 7, Vol 3. pp. 31–38. Retrieved from https://www.mydigitalpublication.com/publication/?i=497397#{"issue_id":497397,"page":32
Robbins, R. (2017). Personal communication.
Seaman, A. M. (2012, December 31). Pediatricians say kids need recess during school. Health News. Retrieved from https://www.reuters.com/article/us-schools-recess/pediatricians-say-kids-need-recess-during-school-idUSBRE8BU02820121231
Selwyn, D. (2010). Following the threads. New York: Peter Lang.
Shulkind, S. B. & Foote, J. (n.d.). Creating a culture of connectedness through middle school advisory programs. Association for Middle Level Education. Retrieved from https://www.amle.org/BrowsebyTopic/WhatsNew/WNDet/TabId/270/ArtMID/888/ArticleID/279/Culture-of-Connectedness-through-Advisory.aspx
Talis, N. (2016, March 15). Census says: Farm to school is booming! National Farm to School Network. Retrieved from http://www.farmtoschool.org/news-and-articles/tag/Healthier_Lunches/
Tedford, H. (2017). Personal communication.
Wood, G. (2004). In Littky, 2004. Big picture: Education is everyone's business. Alexandria, VA: ASCD p. 62.

·10·

IT TAKES A VILLAGE TO CHANGE A VILLAGE

When I think about Sam, my former student whose story I briefly told in the first chapter, I try to think of what would have had to be different for his story to have been less traumatic and more positive. He was dealing with virtually every category of challenge on the list; his family was desperately poor, they were dealing with the current presence of racism and the centuries of racism, discrimination, and genocide that has defined the interactions between native communities and the majority white, European-descended population of the United States. Alcoholism is rampant among many native communities, a consequence of that history, and it was true for Sam's family. He lived in a community overwhelmed by a sense of hopelessness, and it seemed there was no light at the end of his particular tunnel. Add to that poor nutrition, being uprooted several times in his young life, entering new classrooms with low skills and no friends, and it's an overwhelming package. I also want to add that Sam brought many strengths to our classroom and to his life, and his creativity, humor, intelligence (in its many forms), and perseverance have served him well and helped him to travel as far as he has.

While Sam's situation is extreme, there are many others who also struggle with severe issues that compromise their health and well-being. It isn't just Sam. We as teachers also recognize that there is only so much we can do when a child comes to us carrying such a heavy load from outside, and so we assess what we can offer and do what we can, heading home at night wishing we could somehow wave a wand and make the fundamental changes that would leave all children and families healthy.

Given the complex, interconnected, and overwhelming challenges that our families and communities face, it takes a coordinated and cooperative effort among as many parties as possible to make fundamental change. There are actions we can take within our classrooms and within our schools, some of which I have talked about in the previous chapter, but that's not enough. That would not have supported Sam's family to lead healthier and more hopeful lives and would not have offered the family and community the resources they needed to be able to raise their children with a sense of health and hope. This level of change requires communities working together at the governmental, institutional, organizational, community, and personal levels.

Working in Community

When we learn history in school we are often focused on the "great men" who were instrumental in bringing change. Martin Luther King was the Civil Rights movement. George Washington was the American Revolution. Abraham Lincoln was the Civil War. This is a dangerous and limiting approach to history for so many reasons. First among them is that it is inaccurate and incomplete. Second is that it presents the notion that change only happens when a great man comes along to lead the charge, which not only eliminates women from the picture but removes awareness of and appreciation for the organizing and actions done by people throughout communities to make change. Activist and educator Angela Davis talks about the Montgomery Bus Boycott:

> Dominant representations of the Black freedom movement are a discrete series of historical moments largely produced by the 1955 Bus Boycott. And somehow, although Martin Luther King Jr. himself began to emerge to prominence as a consequence of that boycott, he is seen as always already the orator and leader of the civil rights movement.
>
> Even though numbers of books, both scholarly and popular, have been written on the role of women in the 1955 boycott, Dr. King, who was actually invited to be a spokesperson for a movement when he was entirely unknown—the movement had already formed—Dr. King remains the dominant figure. (Davis and Barat, 2016, 65–66)

King was not the movement; the movement was tens of thousands of African-American women, children, and men who chose to act with a unity of purpose against the segregation of Montgomery buses and was part of a history of resistance and struggle going back hundreds of years. It's not that King was insignificant, but that it was the actions of the community working together that brought the change. When "the great man theory" is the lens through which we are taught to look, we are taught to discount the actions of the members of the community, especially the women, and to stay passive until a great man (our prince) comes along to lead us. It is a way of keeping the status quo and is a debilitating message. Change comes through the concerted and coordinated actions of the many, often over time. Skilled leadership is essential, but those leaders are not the full story, and they are not only men. It takes a village to change the village, using the resources or "assets" in that village, perhaps at times working with other villages to create the change they want to be.

As we contemplate the actions we can take to reduce inequality and bring better health in our own time, it seems certain that leadership for this action will not be coming from the current administration. This means that it is up to us to act for our own health and for the health of our communities.

An Asset-Based Approach

An asset-based approach is an approach to community development, to making change by beginning with an assessment of the resources, the assets that exist within the community. This approach, developed by McKnight and Kretzmann, is particularly valuable for those looking to make significant change in communities without large bank accounts or obvious, traditional resources:

> Asset-based community development (ABCD) is a methodology for the sustainable development of communities based on their strengths and potentials. It involves assessing the resources, skills, and experience available in a community; organizing the community around issues that move its members into action; and then determining and taking appropriate action. This method uses the community's own assets and resources as the basis for development; it empowers the people of the community by encouraging them to utilize what they already possess. (McKnight and Kretzmann, 1993)

One of the key features of an asset-based approach is to redefine the resources a community brings, moving beyond a focus on dollars and cents. Leo Hwang, Greenfield Community College Dean of Humanities, talks about an asset-based approach as it pertains to working with community:

> The first thing that comes to mind when people think of traditional assets are the kinds of things people think of when you are writing a will [...] your property, or your bank account, investments, but we are interested in assets beyond those categories, like the skills that people have. When someone has been trained in mediation skills, is a writer and has editing skills, is a website designer, has legal expertise, is adept at keeping books, can repair automobiles, all those are valuable assets. There are also assets that can get lost in between the financial assets and the skills, like when someone has tools, someone has access to parks and buildings, someone has a band saw and a table saw. Once you start making an inventory of all these things and you can almost immediately recognize their potential for connections. So, if one maps or catalogs these assets, it is easier to create connections of combinations of assets that enable possibility. It engenders a feeling that you can create an endeavor right here, and if you have everything you need. [...] It is, of course, still complicated and hard work, but the energy of we can do this is very different than listing all the reasons why we can't. So that's really the power of looking at things that way, starting from a place of assets and possibility. (Hwang, 2018, personal communication)

Schools too often focus on what they don't have, what they can't do. The asset-based approach, as described by Hwang, shifts focus to recognizing the resources that do exist within the community and figuring out how to best take advantage of them.

Working With the School Community

The first place to turn when thinking of school and community is the literal school community, the families who connect to the school as parents of children who attend (or previously attended), the families connected to those who work at the school or who work with programs already connected to the school, and the faculty and staff at the school. Every school community contains a wealth of resources or assets that can be brought to the school to support the learning and health of the students.

Teachers Working With Teachers

Teachers can be each other's best resource, if they can find the time to take advantage of the assets that each brings. This is one of the places that the school structure can support teachers working together by scheduling common planning periods for grade levels. When a common prep period is a daily event for grade-level teams, they can sit together to talk about students, about curricular issues, about challenges they are having in meeting the needs of students. Teachers have different strengths, different experiences, different resources and connections, and ideas about how best to teach certain curriculum, how best to reach particular kinds of learners, and they are likely to be more effective in serving their students when they can share those resources with each other. It may seem an obvious thing to have schedules in common, but it happens way too rarely. Scheduling is complex because there are so many moving parts to fit together, but if the schedule is constructed with the needs of the students as the top priority it can happen more often than it does currently.

This is trickier at the secondary level, since students are with several different teachers a day as they move from subject to subject but structuring common time by grade level, even once or twice a month, allows teachers to talk with each other about the students they share or allows subject area teachers to compare notes and share resources. I don't want to pretend this is easy to arrange given how busy teachers are, but I know having time to talk with colleagues made my teaching more effective, and it allowed us to coordinate what we were doing in our various subject areas so that students were making connections from one subject with another. I worked with an art teacher, for example, when I was teaching about countries in Africa, and he helped students to explore the arts and mask making of some of the people we were studying, and we were able to explore the ways in which the arts and culture intersected with the history they were learning in my classes. At the same time, the students were reading literature from some of those countries in their ELA classes, short stories that offered another lens through which to view the region. It helped the students to connect from one class to another and to make more meaning from what they were studying. This could only happen through the teachers having time to plan together, to coordinate our lessons enough that there was some coherence for the students.

Parents, Families, and Staff

I depended heavily on and benefited from the skills and resources we had in our school communities. In elementary school I was fortunate to have parents and family members who became active participants in our class, sharing their knowledge, skills, and materials with us. There were parents and family members who were in my room on a regular basis, offering help to those who needed extra support in reading or math, helping to organize and drive on field trips, sharing information about their jobs and their hobbies and interests, helping us with art projects, sharing slides of travel or of relatives who lived abroad. Families who had lived in other parts of the country or the world brought us slides and stories of what it was like to grow up and live elsewhere. Their involvement made our experience in the classroom much deeper and more valuable, and their children took pride and comfort in their being with us and honored for their contributions. In addition to our room parents, other parents and school community members came into the room to assist. The involvement of the larger school community helped all of the students to become more connected with the school community, broadening their world and deepening their connection to it.

Community members also became involved in more focused ways on larger projects. When my third-grade classroom was studying homelessness, which I have written about before (Selwyn, 1993), our children became concerned that the children living on the streets would be cold and wanted to do something for them. They decided that they wanted to make quilts to keep at least a couple of kids warm, and when they found out that there was a school for homeless children in Seattle they decided to donate our quilts to a classroom in that school. They had never thought about the fact that homeless children often had to move during a school year and so having a school they could attend no matter where they were staying was an important anchor for them. This sounded like a wonderful idea to me, and I was excited to bring many aspects of quilts to our reading, writing, math, and social studies curriculums, but I had no idea how to make a quilt, much less a quilt large enough to keep twenty-five active eight- and nine-year-olds involved. I found out that there were quilt makers in our school community and they volunteered to come in for a day to share their quilts and to talk about them. When they heard what we were doing, they became regular members of our class; their looms stayed in the classroom and they came in nearly every day for the weeks it took to design and create the quilts. They had connections with fabric stores in town and got those stores to donate the fabric we needed to create two quilts.

Someone else in our community had connections to the local organization that had helped to bring the AIDS quilt to town, and she helped to bring someone from that organization to our classroom with squares from the AIDS quilt, especially a couple of squares memorializing children. It was not an easy session, but the presenters handled the session beautifully and the children came away even more determined to create and deliver their quilts.

The mayor of our city happened to meet one of our students who asked him how the city dealt with homeless people, and when the mayor heard about the work we were doing in class he was so impressed that he visited our classroom and spoke with us about the city's response (or lack of response) to the needs of the city's homeless population, especially during winter. The children asked why the city didn't open up buildings to the homeless when it got cold, and the city now does that. I'm not sure it was because of their questions, but I'm sure it didn't hurt.

I brought in a social worker who was working with homeless teenagers and she not only talked about what it was really like to be homeless and living on the streets, but she brought with her a teenager who was homeless and who talked about what it was like for him. Having a teenager in the classroom who really was homeless brought the issue that much closer to my eight- and nine-year-olds. One of the quiet secrets to our study was that two of our classmates were homeless and the rest of the class did not know it. I talked with them and their families about what we were doing, and they preferred to not share their situation, which remained a secret. A nice, quiet benefit to our study was that we were able to uncover some resources and connections that proved to be helpful to those two families.

My class met with students from the classroom we were donating the quilts to and the children got to spend the afternoon together. My students came to realize that homeless children are children, just like them, who happened to be homeless, which was a powerful learning moment.

This is one example of using the connections within the school community to further the experience of the students and to help them become more grounded and aware of their community and of the ways they could play a role in making it better.

Immigration Stories

Another example involved a project I carried out with my fourth-/fifth-grade students looking at immigration. They were a class of students who were mostly recent immigrants (the ones I talked about in relation to testing), and their families were still very connected with family from their countries of origin. We spent many months collecting stories from each family about the first person from their family to come to Washington State (where we were). Students interviewed their parents or older relatives for those stories, brought in photographs and clothing and artifacts. We interviewed some parents and community members, including some of the instructional assistants who worked in the school. Families sent in stories and books they remembered from their time growing up elsewhere. We created a book of those welcome to Washington stories, featuring the stories of the families represented in our classroom. We could not have done this without the support of the children's families and the willingness of our instructional assistants, who told their own stories and helped to translate some of the stories the families told. I've told some of this story in *Social Studies at the Center* (Lindquist and Selwyn, 2000).

Growing a School Community Garden

A third example involved a whole school effort to create a community garden at the school. Parents and family members from the PTA supported our request to create a garden so that the children could learn about plants and farming by actually creating and maintaining a garden on our grounds. We had to go through steps to get an ok from the school district, but once that happened, the families went to work. They found donations from neighborhood nurseries and construction companies. There were whole school work parties on more than a few Saturdays, where adults and children created the garden space, did the planting and garden maintenance. Neighborhood families maintained the garden over the summer vacation. And when school reopened in the fall, there was some small harvest to share. The students had the opportunity to learn more about the cycle of life, about food and nutrition, and about what goes into producing the food they take for granted at a grocery store or at home. We also came together more as a community, working together on the garden.

Our Day in Court

I held mock trials in my high school U.S. history classes and we had a lawyer or two in the school community who volunteered time with us in helping to understand how trials worked, what the role of the prosecutors, defense attorneys and judges were, and helped the students prepare for their trials. We also got support from the larger community as we prepared to take our mock trials to the King County courthouse. The local branch of the ACLU provided materials about the justice system and provided mock trial samples that informed the work we were doing. A lawyer friend of mine came to class and worked additional hours with those who were going to actually try the case at the courthouse, and an actual King County judge volunteered to be the judge at our trial.

Many of my students had never been in a courthouse, so when we carried out the trial they were a bit in awe, just being in this seat of power. We went through all the steps of the trial, beginning with a bailiff having us all rise when the judge entered. The students learned about how the courts work, the challenge of both presenting arguments clearly and persuasively, and sorting through conflicting information and accounts to discover "the truth," which according to their reflections changed the way they approached what they were reading or hearing.

One other note. The stars of the mock trial were several students who often struggled with the more traditional "read the text and answer the questions" type of educational task. They were also marginal test takers, and I'm sure their standardized test scores were borderline at best. They were extraordinary in the trial. They knew and understood their characters and their story, they stayed in character through the entire trial, and they were effective at arguing their case. One of the prosecuting attorneys was so good at questioning witnesses that the judge said to him, "A., I wish I could get my attorneys to question witnesses the way you do." Another student was missing when the trial was about to begin, and we worried about where she might be. I went out in the hallway and saw her walking slowly toward the courtroom, a small, slow-moving gray-haired figure who shook slightly. She entered the courtroom to gasps from her classmates, who had not seen her in full makeup, and made way for her with a courtesy and respect that reflected her age. She shook on the witness stand and was flawless in telling her account of the events in question.

We could not have offered the students this experience without involvement of the community, and it enriched their school experience. Students who were marginally engaged in their education became passionately engaged in the material related to the trials, both in class and then at the courthouse, and students who had never really found success in the classroom truly shined through this experience.

Natural Helpers: Assets in the School Community

Natural Helpers came out of a concern surrounding teen suicides and depression. The program is based around a simple but profound concept that there are natural helpers within any school community, people who others turn to for support. The key awareness is that these helpers are not always people you'd expect, or people positions such as teachers or counselors. Students are asked (anonymously) to identify those people they turn to when they need support, and often their choices surprise everyone, including those who are identified. They might include guidance counselors or coaches, but they might also include people who work in the lunchroom, or custodians, or students who are all but invisible to much of the school but are identified as good friends who are always there to help. The program then offers recognition, and then training and support to those who have been identified, so that they are more able to do what they are already doing, which is to help others and to be recognized and appreciated for what they do.

The program still exists; I found reference to it under the title Peer to Peer, and it is being used around the country. It is another example of redefining or recognizing the assets that exist within a community and supporting those assets.

Acting Together

I want to highlight two more example of a school community working together. The first is to take a brief look at the wildcat strikes that took place this school year (2018) in four states. The second is to look at actions taken at one public school in Seattle that soon spread across the city and then across the country.

Teacher Walkouts

Teachers across the country have begun reaching out to each other as they have not done for many, many years, recognizing that there is only so much they can do alone. Wildcat strikes in "red states" such as West Virginia, Oklahoma, Arizona, and Kentucky were a consequence of those states and the federal government enacting policies that were starving the schools. Olivia Morris, a West Virginia teacher, talked about what led to the West Virginia teachers walking out:

> Healthcare was bad, the pay was bad, the working conditions were bad [...] You've got too many kids in the classroom. It's the same issues that we see across the country and across the world and we saw that people were already really fed up and they wanted action. (Peterson, 2018)

Teachers were moved to strike because of the poor pay and benefits, but also because of the ways in which the underfunding of the schools was hurting children. There were concerns about school safety, about inadequate materials, outdated textbooks, overcrowded classrooms due to teacher shortages, and an unwillingness of those in state education and in the legislature to listen. Their students were suffering, they were being shortchanged in their education, and the teachers had reached a point where they could not let that continue.

Two things are of paramount importance here. One is that these strikes happened because the school workers stood together, recognizing that their acting together was their power, their strength, and that as much as the state might huff and puff, without teachers in the classroom schools could not operate, and there could not be business as usual.

The second is that when they acted, the community stood with them. The community knew that teachers were acting in their own interests, wanting fairer salaries and pensions and the like, but that they were also acting in the interests of the children who were being cheated out of a quality education and of the opportunity to live healthy and productive lives by the underfunding of schools. The teachers and community came together in common cause, and their actions forced movement by the legislatures in the respective states. When the governments tried to separate the educators from the community, saying the teachers should go back for the sake of the children (the line they always use), the teachers and community stood firm. And they won. The concessions they secured were admittedly modest, but they were a small step closer to full funding and a giant step closer to becoming a politically formidable movement.

These actions have obvious short-term benefits, with teachers getting their small raises and a commitment for better school funding, but there are longer term consequences that are equally important. The teachers have seen that they do not have to stand alone, in isolation, feeling powerless. They can reach out, through their unions or in spite of their unions, to connect with each other to work in community for change. In addition, their students are seeing the very best modeling they could see, adults standing up for what they believe and taking action, taking a risk to make things better. It is what we hope they will do throughout their lives.

Doing Nothing Is a Political Act

What teachers have modeled all too often is the notion that even if they don't like what is happening there is nothing they can do. Many teachers say they don't want to get involved with politics and that they just want to teach their children. What they are beginning to learn is that by doing nothing they are engaging in a political action, allowing the status quo to continue, and that their inaction is hurting their children and public education. These strike actions have demonstrated that by acting, they are serving their children by bringing about needed funding for education and by modeling the possibilities of acting with others to make change.

Consider the brief scenario I shared in the introduction about my conversations with colleagues who were complaining about testing. When I suggested we stand together and not give the tests, my colleagues could not conceive of taking such a public and political action, afraid of what might happen. More teachers are now closer to realizing that they do have power and a responsibility to stand up for their students and for their profession and that together they can act to make things better.

Black Lives Matter in Schools

The second example of teachers and the community working together comes from Seattle. In September of 2016 the community at John Muir elementary, in South Seattle, held an event called "Black Men Uniting to Change the Narrative." The event was the idea of Muir family and student advocate DeShawn Jackson, who said he wanted "to show our students that our black men weren't what they see and hear on TV and in the news" (Corn, 2018). Dozens of African-American men welcomed students into the school on that day, African drummers drummed, and teachers, wearing Black Lives Matter tee shirts, taught about racism in their classrooms.

The event came after months of the staff studying the politics of privilege and race and was supported by the parents and the school's administration. The school population at Muir is nearly fifty percent African-American, nearly eighty percent students of color, and the staff was committed to sending a positive message to all students to counter what students were seeing through media. They wanted their students to feel safe and supported and valued and having this strong gathering of black men to celebrate them was part of it. They also wanted to make sure that the education the students were getting included an honest, age-appropriate study of issues including race, class, and privilege. The staff felt it important that their education made them more aware, more complete in their understanding of why things are the way they are and to become aware of allies in the community who are working to make things fairer and more just.

The event was nearly cancelled; in fact, it was cancelled by the Seattle School District after a bomb threat was called in, but after bomb sniffing dogs found nothing, the school decided to open and to hold the event, refusing to be intimidated or stopped by the threats of white supremacists.

From there, the movement spread across the city. Teachers from Muir talked with members of Social Equality Educators (S.E.E.), a rank and file organization of union educators, and eventually that group voted to have a district-wide action, to follow up what had happened at Muir. They agreed that on October 19, teachers across the entire school district would (voluntarily) wear Black Lives Matter tee shirts and spend the day teaching lessons about racism. The S.E.E. brought a resolution to the Seattle Education Association, the union representing all of Seattle's teachers, looking for support for the action. S.E.E. also developed a three-point policy proposal that would serve as an ongoing campaign to support Black Lives Matter in schools and aid in the struggle against institutional racism:

1. Support ethnic studies in all schools.
2. Replace zero-tolerance discipline with restorative justice practices.
3. De-track classes within the schools to undo the racial segregation that is reinforced by tracking. (Au and Hagopian, 2017)

The union voted to support the action, and additional support also came from the Seattle chapter of the NAACP, from parent groups, and, surprisingly, from the Seattle School District administration.

Muir parent and University of Washington professor Wayne Au sent a letter out requesting support from university professors around the country and in a couple of days had more than 250 professors supporting the action, and word of the action became national news.

The day of celebration in October was a success; teachers in all schools in the district were wearing Black Lives Matter tee shirt and teaching about racism and privilege. The coalition of teachers, parents, unions, organizations such as the NAACP and the school district administration had joined together to make a strong political statement against racism, against white supremacy, and for justice and quality education for all. That movement has continued and grown, to where this year (2018) there was a week-long focus on race and privilege in several cities across the country.

> From February 5–9, Black Lives Matter shirts will fill classrooms from Seattle to LA, Chicago, Detroit, New York City, Philadelphia, Washington, DC, Boston, and more, along with history lessons on institutional racism.

> "This is a growing movement to sever the school-to-prison pipeline," said organization spokesperson and Garfield High School ethnic studies teacher Jesse Hagopian, "and to make sure the curriculum that we have in our classrooms uplift our black students and give them lessons they need to help be part of the struggle to undo institutional racism." (Corn, 2018)

This action began through the collective concern, study, and organizing of the faculty at Muir. They came together out of common concern about racism, in the larger society, in the school district, and in the community. They centered their action in their school, bringing in people from the community to make the event happen. Their actions inspired other actions, across town and then across the country.

The Seattle Education Association posted links to resources for those interested in teaching about Black Lives Matter and other race-related issues. You can find those resources at this address:

> http://www.seattlewea.org/center-for-race-equity/Black%20Lives%20Matter%20Week%20Resources/

School Boards

One of the places that school districts and the community come together is through school boards or school committees (as they are sometimes known). These boards are comprised of a small group of adults from the community (anywhere from three to ten) who are elected to their positions for short terms, though they can be reelected and serve for many years. Their role is to help set policy, to oversee the operations of the district, to deal with the budget and capital decisions, and to hire the superintendent and other district-level positions. What they do is enormously consequential, beginning with the hiring of the superintendent and other upper level district administration, and their decisions on policy can have enormous consequences. Here are two brief examples.

The school district in Wake County North Carolina had achieved racial integration through busing, through having urban and suburban children attending the schools together. That policy was supported by the school board. That policy was changed when four new board members, supported by an organized group determined to take over the school board, were elected in 2009. Their election moved the board to a very conservative majority. Fewer than eight percent of potential voters went to the polls for that vote, and the new five to four majority ended the racial diversity program that had been district policy for years before, despite the overwhelming support for the program from the school community and from the city.

A similar story holds true in Golden Colorado. In 2009 three new board members were elected to the five-person board, giving them an instant majority, and with that majority they turned the school district policy upside down.

> The Douglas County board hired a new superintendent, ended bargaining with the teachers' union and, perhaps most controversially, approved a voucher plan using public funds to help students—even those from wealthy families—attend private schools. The Colorado Supreme Court rejected the voucher program this summer, but the district is appealing that decision to the U.S. Supreme Court. (Fish, 2015)

Voter turnout was low, only around thirty-three percent, and those who showed up have made a significant difference in the lives of the children and educators in that district. Those who show up for the next election will also have the opportunity to make a significant difference in the lives of the children and educators in the district.

School boards set policy, and often three people living in a county can change a policy despite it being endorsed by a majority of educators and families. Because they are not often high-profile races, voter turnout is often very low, which means that a well-organized campaign coupled with voter turnout can result in a drastic change in district policy, seemingly overnight.

Three lessons to take from this: First, find candidates who care about the health and well-being of children, who value diversity and child-centered education. Second, organize to support those candidates, to educate the public about why their vision of education will best serve the children and the community. And third, organize and work for voter turnout. With low voter turnout, every vote matters.

Once the School Board Is Elected

It is important to remember, with all due respect, that since many if not most of the people serving on school boards are not educators they may or may not fully understand the issues with which they are dealing. I do not mean this as a slight or critique of those on the board who are volunteering their time and who care about children and about education. Their lack of knowledge about how schools work or how times have changed since they were in school may lead them, with the best intentions, to be voting on issues while being relatively uninformed or misinformed. That suggests a level of community involvement that helps to respectfully "educate" the members of the school board. Support them through conversations and through sharing materials, articles, data, and stories. Show up and make public comment at school board meetings so that they hear from the public. Those few voices who show up can make a significant difference, at times alerting school board members to issues or points of view they otherwise would not have considered. It does not take many members of the community to make a difference. When the local school district was considering whether to hire additional Community Resource Officers (police) in the schools following the Parkland shooting, students and teachers came to the school board meeting and said they did not want the officers, they wanted the resources used to hire more counselors and others who worked with the students. The board listened to them.

Involving the Larger Community

Hernandez et al (2013) note that

> the literature in the field emphasizes "healthy communities" as a process, not a status. A healthy community is one that seeks to improve the health of its citizens by putting health high on the social and political agenda. Healthy communities are about the process that enables people to improve their health through applying the concepts and principles of health promotion at the local level. (Hernandez et al, 2013)

Real, sustainable change takes time. Patience has never been the strong point of the American makeup, and with the twenty-four-hour news cycle and the demand for instant satisfaction, many politicians are leery of taking on an effort that might take years to produce recognizable change. Once again, this means that it is up to us on the local level, in our neighborhoods and communities, to take the small, constant steps that change requires, steps that move much slower than do headlines.

Fundamental, lasting change requires addressing underlying causes, determinants of health, which are complicated and often inextricably bound together. Hernandez says that

> Communities *become healthier* (emphasis in original) as people are empowered to develop critical awareness concerning the avoidable causes of ill-health and are

> prepared to change attitudes and behavior concerning their own lifestyles. Communities *become healthier* when their members increase the control over the factors that relate local conditions to the "social determinants" of their own health. (Hernandez et al, 2013)

There are an increasing number of examples of communities beginning to work together to address these fundamental needs, not only on a short-term basis but also on a more fundamental level with an eye toward real solutions.

I will share three examples of the community working together to make change in Franklin County, Massachusetts (where we now live) because they represent efforts being made by people throughout this community that are similar to work being done in other communities and regions as well. They are based on models that can be replicated and adapted to fit the population and needs of each community or region, and they involve both short-term and long-term actions that depend more on people and organizations working together than they do on money.

I am not presenting them as perfect, nor as "the answer," the model that others should follow, but as examples of interdisciplinary, coordinated efforts one community is making to make change. There are hundreds if not thousands of examples from around the country that could also serve as inspiration for what is possible when a community decides to stop waiting for the great men at the top to finally hear them and to act.

Community Health Improvement Plan for Franklin County and North Quabbin

The Community Health Improvement Plan (CHIP) program being carried out throughout Franklin County, Massachusetts, is coordinated by the Franklin Regional Council of Governments, or FRCOG. This effort brings together the resources, organizations, agencies, and institutions of the Franklin County region to bring what they call an evidence-based approach to improving the health of the county. They were initially supported by funding by the Robert Wood Johnson Foundation (RWJF) and have relied heavily on research carried out by RWJF, which has done county-wide assessments of health across the United States. With this data to guide their actions, the CHIP program has focused on addressing what the research shows to be the major determinants of health in our community. The vision and mission statements put out by CHIP read as follows:

Franklin County/North Quabbin CHIP

VISION All residents of Franklin County and the North Quabbin Region have the opportunity to pursue healthy lifestyles and achieve social, emotional, physical, and spiritual well-being; and to participate in shaping the systems that affect their health.

MISSION With this vision in mind, we intend for this Community Health Improvement Planning process to provide a clear plan that:

- identifies priority health needs and disparities and the factors that contribute to them;
- builds on our strengths by identifying current resources in the community to address priority health issues;
- identifies the most effective strategies for addressing the priority health needs;
- reduces gaps and duplication in services; and
- increases our collective ability to secure resources to improve health in our region.

The CHIP effort has brought together a wide range of community resources, focused on identifying and acting together to improve the health of the community. Organizations in this effort include:

Baystate Franklin Medical Center; Clinical & Support Options (CSO); Communities That Care Coalition; Community Action of the Franklin, Hampshire, and North Quabbin Regions; Community Health Center of Franklin County; Franklin Regional Council of Governments (FRCOG); Franklin Regional Housing and Redevelopment Authority; FRCOG's Mass in Motion Program; FRCOG's Transportation Planning Program; Greenfield Health Department; LifePath North Quabbin Community Coalition Opioid Task Force of Franklin County and North Quabbin; United Way of Franklin County

They used the data from RWJF to identify ten key health issues in the Franklin County/North Quabbin region, identified policies and programs with the strongest likelihood of success, and then made decisions about what actions to take over the next three years (2017–2020) based on their assessment of what was already happening in the region, what gaps they could identify, and what strategies were not yet being enacted.

The data from RWJF broke down the determinants of health in ways that mirror data I found from other sources, a mix of the physical environment (air and water quality), social and economic factors (community safety, family and social support, income, employment, education), clinical care (access to care, quality of care), and health behaviors (tobacco use, diet and exercise, alcohol and drug use, sexual activity).

Guided by this data, the CHIP (Franklin/North Quabbin) program is currently engaged in several actions in each of those four areas, either continuing programs that have been making a difference or beginning new ones to address a concern that has not yet been addressed. Here are a few of the action strategies they are focused on for this three-year period:

Health Behaviors: Diabetes prevention; substance abuse prevention curriculum in schools; increasing access to green spaces and parks; school nutrition standards; healthy food bank initiatives; family drug court implementation and evaluation; tobacco cessation groups.

Clinical Care: Clarifying the definition of and standardizing the training of community health workers; fluoride varnish; chronic disease self-management programs.

Social and economic factors: nurturing families' group-based parenting classes; paid family leave; increasing the minimum wage; fair share amendment (the millionaire's tax).

Physical environment: Housing first, housing rehab and loans; increased public transportation/on-demand transport.

Most of these actions are focused on the local level, but a few of them, particularly in the social and economic factors category, are part of state-wide efforts to change fundamental policy related to health and well-being across the entire state.

This is a wide-ranging, challenging effort that looks at both taking preventative steps and responding to current needs and threats to health. The various participants in the effort meet regularly to plan and assess. Their current effort is conceived of as a three-year plan, recognizing that it takes time to make change. They have seen positive changes as a result of some of their action steps, and others have not been in operation long enough to assess. They will reassess in three years and make changes, based on those assessments, as they form a plan to determine the focus for the following three years.

Communities That Care/Collective Impact Model

Communities that Care in Franklin County uses an approach that has been called "Collective Impact," a focused, coordinated effort that brings together many key players in the community. Kramer et al describe the five conditions of Collective Impact:

> Common Agenda: All participants have a shared vision for change including a common understanding of the problem and a joint approach to solving it through agreed upon actions.

Shared Measurement: Collecting data and measuring results consistently across all participants ensures efforts remain aligned and participants hold each other accountable.

Mutually reinforcing Activities: Participant activities must be differentiated while still being coordinated through a mutually reinforcing plan of action.

Continuous Communication: Consistent and open communication is needed across the many players to build trust, assure mutual objectives, and create common motivation.

Backbone Support: Creating and managing collective impact requires a separate organization with staff and a specific set of skills to serve as the backbone for the entire initiative and coordinate participating organizations and agencies. (Stanford Social Innovation Review, Channeling Change: Making Collective Impact Work, 2012)

The Franklin County Communities that Care coalition works according to this model and now coordinates more than 200 representatives from social service agencies, the district attorney's office, schools, police departments, youth serving agencies, faith-based organizations, local elected officials, local businesses, media, parents, and youth.

The group originally came together in 2002 over concerns about teen drinking and drug use to focus their efforts on specific targeted actions designed to reduce risky behaviors and to increase healthy ones. They were trained in and followed the national Communities That Care community planning system, which was developed by Seattle-based researchers David Hawkins and Richard Catalano. The model guides communities through surveying local youth to determine the specific local needs and then adopting tested and effective programs to address these needs. Following this model, the Franklin County coalition surveyed local youth in the ten school districts within the region so that their approaches to addressing youth health issues are most likely to be appropriate for the Franklin County region and population.

Their results have been impressive. There have been significant and substantial reductions in teen binge drinking and alcohol use, teen smoking, and teen marijuana use.

Kat Allen oversees the prevention efforts and Rachel Stoler coordinates the nutrition and physical activity part of the effort. Allen talked about the project.

I work to coordinate the coalition's work on substance use prevention, and Rachel oversees our work in improving nutrition and physical activity. We are really focused on building protection and moving towards health. We conduct an annual teen health survey to understand what health-behavior choices local kids are making, as well as what risk factors and protective factors in the community, the schools, and in families are contributing to healthy—or unhealthy—choices. Based on what we learn from the survey, we support prevention programs and strategies—in the schools, in the community, and in families—that have been tested and found to be effective in addressing the specific local needs. Some of our core strategies include helping the schools to implement evidence-based substance use prevention curricula in health classes, supporting school nurses in having formalized one-on-one conversations about substance use with each high school student, working with towns to adopt zoning, advertising, and other policies that support health, providing evidence-based parent education programs and information for parents, etc.

We convene several workgroups, including a Regional Schools Health Task Force which meets monthly and includes representatives from each of the nine local school districts. All of the local schools participate in the survey, and the Regional School Health Task Force oversees and implements the survey, as well as helps to link the other coalition workgroups (such as the Parent Education Workgroup and the Policy and Practice Change Workgroup) to the schools. A lot of great information gets shared between schools at these meetings. (Allen, 2018, personal communication)

Rachel Stoler heads the effort focused on improving healthy behaviors. Recently they carried out an assessment of the nutrition programs in every school district in the region. They hired a person to observe mealtime in schools in every district, to note what foods they offered, how they presented them to the students, how they communicated about the foods and about what good nutrition looks like, and to identify the challenges the districts faced in improving the nutrition they could offer to their students.

Food managers from all of the districts came together to hear a summary of the report, with the consultant highlighting some best practices she felt worth sharing to the whole group. Each food service manager also received a detailed report pertaining to her particular district, which will help her to assess what is being most effective and where she might make changes.

This model, of supporting the community to come together to take targeted action, informed by data is typical of the Collective Impact approach, and the results have been positive.

Community Development Corporation

Franklin County is the second poorest county in Massachusetts and is mostly composed of isolated hill towns and a few valley towns such as Greenfield, the county seat. Many of the towns in this area were once mill towns, running on cheaply available water power, but the mills and factories are largely gone and many of the dollars and jobs they once generated have gone with them. The Community Development Corporation is a regional effort to generate and support small, local businesses that help to provide income to county residents, a tax base to support schools and services in the towns, jobs for families living in the area and that help to protect and preserve the environment, which in turn is part of what sustains the economy through attracting tourists.

Working together to support diverse economic development may not necessarily seem like it is a community action in support of health, but as we have seen elsewhere in the book economic inequality and poverty play significant roles in the health of a community. If people have sustainable jobs, good employment that will help them to feed their families, to maintain homes, and to pay their taxes, the entire community benefits.

John Waite, director of the Franklin County Community Development Corporation, talks about the work the CDC does to support and sustain small businesses throughout Franklin County:

> We started in 1979, factories had closed or were closing, people had talents and skills but had no place to work [...] One of our goals is job creation, business creation; if you can get more mid-sized businesses paying taxes that's certainly going to help. Another one of our goals is to maximize community control over our future economic destiny and more local businesses that grow here, hire people here, and stay here are the key, instead of letting multi-national corporations dictate the economy. (Waite, 2018, personal communication)

Part of what the CDC does is to help companies make connections, to support each other for the benefit of both companies and the town. Their work in supporting agriculture and small farms is an example of that.

The CDC is coordinating with the schools, with organizations such as Mass in Motion, that look to get local produce into the schools so that farmers benefit, and children benefit from having good, nutritious food.

Waite adds that "the other connection that is important for health is that local/regional sized food businesses tend to use more real food, less preservatives and sweeteners. So in addition to jobs, which enable residents to make healthier choices, we help make sure those healthier choices actually exist."

Another feature of the CDC is to help new businesses get started. They help prospective entrepreneurs to develop a solid business plan, help them to develop a realistic financial plan, provide loans, and support them once they actually go into business. They make loans to more than one hundred businesses at a time, which means they are supporting a wide swath of the economy in Franklin County. When a business is successful, the entire community benefits.

The combination of helping businesses develop a solid plan, making loans, and supporting businesses to connect with other businesses and with the schools (for example) means that there are more people working, which supports families, raises the tax base, and helps to maintain local control over our economy, all of which contribute to the health of the community.

Working at the State and National Level

The organizing work taking place in communities is crucial to making change, especially during times when the federal government and the states are not willing or able to offer much help, but there is also much to be done to make change at the state and federal level and ways that communities can play a role in bringing about that change. This work ranges from taking an active part in political campaigns for candidates who support issues that bring more health and well-being to the community to working on state-wide campaigns and legislation related to issues such as school funding, single-payer health care, community green banking, raising the minimum wage, a sustainable energy policy based on renewable resources such as wind and solar, and the millionaires tax in Massachusetts, which would add a four percent tax on incomes above a million dollars to bring additional funding for schools and transportation. Despite the present climate that makes change at the federal or state level supporting health unlikely, it is still important to keep pushing, keep organizing, and coordinating efforts to support the necessary policy changes, even while knowing that they won't happen today. Or tomorrow.

There are many ways that communities can work together to support their populations, and as there are diverse social, economic, health care, and educational determinants to contribute to health, there is a need for and room for all of these efforts. The examples I've highlighted are efforts of one community to work together, assessing their situation and needs, and planning together, making best use of their assets and resources to work together in targeted ways to make a difference. They are realistic enough to know that what they are doing won't solve everything, but their actions do make a difference, and it makes those acting together a stronger, more connected community more willing to take future steps together.

References

Allen, K. (2018). Personal communication.

Au, W. & Hagopian, J. (2017, Fall). How one elementary school sparked a citywide movement to make black students' lives matter. Rethinking Schools. Retrieved from https://www.rethinkingschools.org/articles/how-one-elementary-school-sparked-a-citywide-movement-to-make-black-students-lives-matter

Corn, S. (2018, January 30). Seattle educators, students primed for "Black Lives Matter at School" week. South Seattle Herald. Retrieved from https://southseattleemerald.com/2018/01/30/seattle-educators-students-primed-for-black-lives-matter-at-achool-week/

Davis, A. & Barat, F. (2016). Freedom is a constant struggle: Ferguson, Palestine, and the foundations of a movement. Chicago: Haymarket.

Fish, S. (2015). School board recall vote in Colorado could have national implications. Al Jazeera America. Retrieved from http://america.aljazeera.com/articles/2015/10/30/school-board-recall-colorado.html

Hernandez, L., Lawrence, R. S., & Pronk, N. P. (2013, February). An integrated framework for assessing the value of community-based prevention: A report of the Institute of Medicine. Preventing Chronic Disease 10(2): E22. Retrieved from https://www.researchgate.net/publication/235628290_An_Integrated_Framework_for_Assessing_the_Value_of_Community-Based_Prevention_A_Report_of_the_Institute_of_MedicineCite this publication

Hwang, L. (2018). Personal communication.

Kramer, J., Kania, M., & Hanleybrown, F. (2012). Channeling change: Making collective impact work. Stanford Social Innovation Review. Retrieved from https://ssir.org/articles/entry/channeling_change_making_collective_impact_work

Lindquist, T. & Selwyn, D. (2000). Social studies at the center. Portsmouth, NH: Heinemann.

McKnight, J. L. & Kretzmann, J. P. (1993). Asset based community development. Revolvy. Retrieved from https://www.revolvy.com/main/index.php?s=Asset-based+community+development

Peterson, R. (2018, Spring). The teacher uprising of 2018. Rethinking Schools. Retrieved from https://www.rethinkingschools.org/articles/the-teacher-uprising-of-2018

Selwyn, D. (1993). Living history in the classroom. Tucson: Zephyr.

Waite, J. (2018). Personal communication.

CONCLUSION

What Will We Do?

A Unitarian Minister told this story from the Masai as he led into his sermon, and it seems to sum up much of what I've been trying to say in this book. It's been making the rounds of the internet, so you may have seen it.

> AND HOW ARE THE CHILDREN?
> By Patrick T O'Neill
> Among the most accomplished and fabled tribes of Africa, no tribe was considered to have warriors more fearsome or more intelligent than the mighty Masai. It is perhaps surprising, then, to learn the traditional greeting that passed between Masai warriors: "Kasserian Ingera," one would always say to another. It means, "And how are the children?"
>
> It is still the traditional greeting among the Masai, acknowledging the high value that the Masai always place on their children's well-being. Even warriors with no children of their own would always give the traditional answer, "All the children are well." Meaning, of course, that peace and safety prevail, that the priorities of protecting the young, the powerless, are in place. That Masai society has not forgotten its reason for being, its proper functions and responsibilities. "All the children are well" means that life is good. It means that the daily struggles for existence do not preclude proper caring for their young. (O'Neill, 2018)

"How are the children?" is a profound and troubling question because we know that at the moment the children are not well. I've presented that unhappy news throughout these pages and identified some reasons why this is so. I've also shared some better news: that people and organizations around the country are finding ways to collaborate, to focus their energies on improving the health and well-being of their children and their communities. The good news is that we have the resources we need to make changes that will leave us healthier and happier. We can rededicate ourselves to the notion of the common good, to putting the well-being of our community over the lure of short-term profits enjoyed by a few and paid for by the many. We can demand that our government represent us rather than serve those who are buying their loyalty. We can make clear that it is not healthy behavior to have some become healthier by having others become less healthy. We can hold the question, "How are the children?" in our awareness and use it as a means by which we assess the health of our schools, our communities, and our society. If our children are not fine, then we are not meeting our responsibilities to them, or to the larger society, which depends on our children being healthy in order to sustain themselves and the society into the future.

It is a question of will. Do we have the will to stand up, to stand together to make change? I've been rereading the *Memories of Fire* trilogy by Eduardo Galeano. This amazing trilogy is a history of the Americas, with a particular focus on Central and South America, and Galeano documents, in the most elegant prose, the invasion, colonizing, and plundering of the many countries of the Americas. He also celebrates the resistance of peoples of the Americas to those invasions, the willingness of those of modest means to stand up to the corporate and military power of the invaders, and to keep their cultures, their spirits, their passions alive. It is that celebration of resistance that gives me hope and reminds that we are many, and this is our home. We have the most at stake here, because we are talking about our children, our land, our air, our water, our lives.

We have a choice to make, about whether to allow their greed and their lust for power and profit to continue to destroy our health and our democracy, or whether we will stand together to say no to them and yes to our health and well-being, and to our children. How are the children? They will be well if we stand for and with them.

References

O'Neill, P. T. (2018). And how are the children? Unitarian Universalist Association. Retrieved from https://www.uua.org/worship/words/reading/and-how-are-the-children

INDEX

C

D

E

F

G

H

I

J

K

L

M

N

O

P

R

S

T

U

V

W

Y

Z

COUNTERPOINTS

Studies in Criticality

General Editor
Shirley R. Steinberg

Counterpoints publishes the most compelling and imaginative books being written in education today. Grounded on the theoretical advances in criticalism, feminism, and postmodernism in the last two decades of the twentieth century, Counterpoints engages the meaning of these innovations in various forms of educational expression. Committed to the proposition that theoretical literature should be accessible to a variety of audiences, the series insists that its authors avoid esoteric and jargonistic languages that transform educational scholarship into an elite discourse for the initiated. Scholarly work matters only to the degree it affects consciousness and practice at multiple sites. Counterpoints' editorial policy is based on these principles and the ability of scholars to break new ground, to open new conversations, to go where educators have never gone before.

For additional information about this series or for the submission of manuscripts, please contact:

Shirley R. Steinberg
c/o Peter Lang Publishing, Inc.
29 Broadway, 18th floor
New York, New York 10006

To order other books in this series, please contact our Customer Service Department:

(800) 770-LANG (within the U.S.)
(212) 647-7706 (outside the U.S.)
(212) 647-7707 FAX

Or browse online by series:

www.peterlang.com

www.ingramcontent.com/pod-product-compliance
Ingram Content Group UK Ltd.
Pitfield, Milton Keynes, MK11 3LW, UK
UKHW020841290926
15470UKWH00004B/1479

9 781433 161636